DISCOVERING NATURAL CURES ACROSS CULTURES

A JOURNEY THROUGH HERBAL HEALING TRADITIONS WORLDWIDE

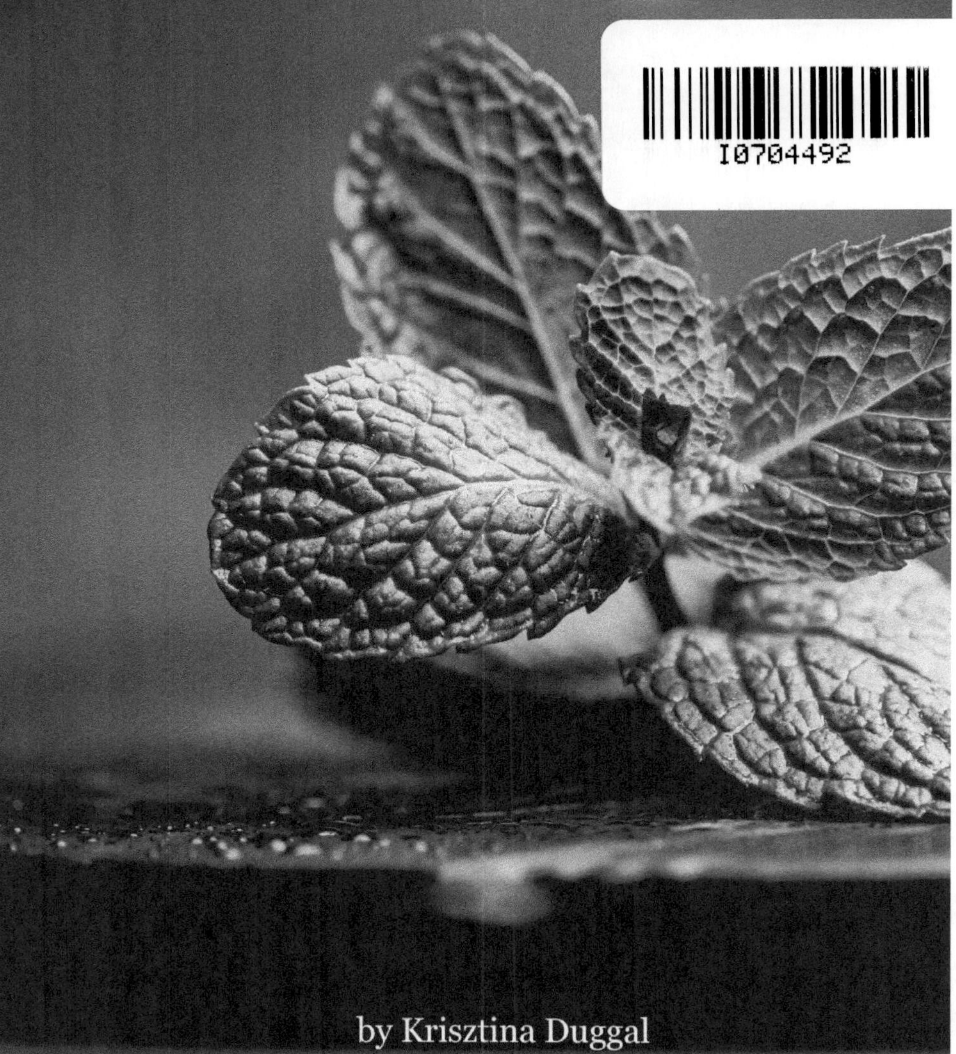

by Krisztina Duggal

KRISZTINA DUGGAL

Discovering Natural Cures Across Cultures

A Journey through herbal healing traditions Worldwide

Contents

1

Introduction

Herbal remedies have been used for centuries to cure various ailments and
diseases across the globe. From ancient civilizations to modern times, herbs
have played a significant role in traditional medicine, offering a natural and
effective way to promote health and well-being. This overview guide
takes you on a journey to explore the diverse world of herbal remedies,
highlighting the unique practices and traditions of various cultures and
regions.

Herbal knowledge has been meticulously documented in ancient texts across various civilizations. In China, the legendary Shen Nong Ben Cao Jing, dating back to the Han dynasty, is one of the earliest known compilations of medicinal plants and their uses. Similarly, the Indian Ayurveda system, with texts like the Charaka Samhita and Sushruta Samhita, offers extensive documentation on herbal remedies and treatment methods. In the Mediterranean, the ancient Greeks and Romans relied on texts such as Dioscorides' De Materia Medica, which cataloged numerous herbs and their applications. These early works form the cornerstone of herbal medicine, encapsulating centuries of empirical wisdom that have guided healers across generations.

Herbalism, the practice of using plants and plant extracts to promote health and wellness, has a rich and diverse history that spans thousands of years. It has played a significant role in the development of medicine and has been used to treat a wide range of diseases.

2

Exploring the Ancient Roots of Herbal Medicine and its Evolution Across Civilizations

Early Beginnings: The Use of Herbs in Ancient Cultures.

The use of herbs in medicine dates back to ancient times, with evidence of herbal remedies being used in civilizations such as Egypt, China, and Greece. In these cultures, herbs were often used in combination with other treatments, such as surgery and spiritual rituals, to treat a wide range of ailments.

In ancient Egypt, for example, herbs were used to treat a variety of conditions, including fever, rheumatism and skin conditions. The Ebers Papyrus, an ancient Egyptian medical text, contains a list of herbal remedies that were used to treat a range of illnesses, including eye infections, wounds and digestive problems.

In ancient China, herbal medicine was an integral part of traditional Chinese medicine, which emphasized the balance of yin and yang and the flow of qi (life energy) in the body. Chinese herbal medicine was used to treat a wide range of conditions, including fever, rheumatism, and digestive problems.

The Golden Age of Herbalism: The Middle Ages and the Renaissance

The Middle Ages and the Renaissance saw a resurgence in the use of herbal medicine, with the development of new herbal remedies and the establishment of herbal medicine as a distinct branch of medicine. During this period, herbalists such as Hildegard of Bingen and John Gerard wrote extensively on the use of herbs in medicine and their works became influential in the development of herbal medicine.

In the 16th century, the publication of the "Herball" by John Gerard, a comprehensive guide to the use of herbs in medicine, marked the beginning of a new era in herbalism. The "Herball" contained descriptions of over 1,000 herbs and their uses, and it became a standard reference work for herbalists and physicians.

The Age of Exploration and the Discovery of New Herbs

The Age of Exploration, which began in the 15th century, saw the discovery of new herbs and the introduction of exotic plants from around the world. This period marked a significant shift in the practice of herbalism, as herbalists began to use new and unfamiliar plants in their remedies. The discovery of new herbs and the development of new herbal remedies were facilitated by the establishment of trade routes and the exchange of knowledge between different cultures.

Trade routes played a pivotal role in the diffusion of herbal knowledge between cultures. The Silk Road, for instance, was more than just a conduit for silk and spices; it facilitated the exchange of medicinal plants and practices between Asia, the Middle East, and Europe. This intercontinental trade enabled the introduction of exotic herbs into new regions, expanding the pharmacopeias of many cultures. The introduction of ginger and turmeric from India to the Arab world and eventually to Europe is a testament to how trade influenced herbal medicine's growth. Such exchanges enriched local healing traditions and fostered a broader understanding of plant-based therapies.

The 19th and 20th Centuries: The Rise of Modern Herbalism

The 19th and 20th centuries saw the rise of modern herbalism, with the development of new herbal remedies and the establishment of herbal medicine as a distinct branch of medicine.

In the late 19th century, the discovery of the alkaloids and glycosides in plants led to the development of new herbal remedies, such as digitalis and quinine. In the 20th century, the development of new herbal remedies continued, with the discovery of new plant compounds.

The 21st Century: The Revival of Herbalism

In recent years, there has been a renewed interest in herbalism, with the development of new herbal remedies. The revival of herbalism has been driven by a growing awareness of the importance of natural and holistic approaches to health and wellness, as well as the increasing recognition of the potential benefits of herbal medicine.

In the modern era, there has been a concerted effort to integrate traditional herbal practices into established healthcare systems. Countries like China and India have maintained robust traditional medicine sectors alongside conventional medical practices. In China, Traditional Chinese Medicine (TCM) is officially recognized and integrated into the national health policy, with hospitals offering both herbal and allopathic treatments.

India's Ministry of AYUSH promotes Ayurveda, Yoga, Unani, Siddha, and Homeopathy within the healthcare framework. This dual approach allows for a more holistic treatment paradigm, recognizing the value of millennia-old practices in addressing contemporary health issues.

3

Mesopotamia

Early Evidence of Herbalism in Mesopotamia

The use of medicinal herbs in Mesopotamia dates back to ancient times, with evidence of their use found in the earliest known medical texts, such as the "Hittite Medical Texts" and the "Yale Culinary Tablet". These texts provide valuable insights into the types of herbs used, their properties, and the diseases and ailments they were used to treat. The Mesopotamians believed that the gods had created the herbs to heal the sick, and as such, they were revered and used with great care.

The Edwin Smith Papyrus, which is one of the oldest known medical texts, contains a collection of medical prescriptions and treatments for various conditions, including skin conditions such as eczema and acne. The papyrus also describes the use of herbs such as myrrh, cedar, and cypress to treat wounds and skin infections. It contains over 700 prescriptions and treatments for various conditions. The papyrus also describes the use of herbs such as chamomile, lavender and thyme.

Medicinal Uses of Herbs in Mesopotamia

The ancient Mesopotamians were known for their advanced understanding of medicine and their use of medicinal herbs to treat a wide range of diseases. The region's unique climate and geography allowed for a diverse range of flora to thrive, providing a rich source of medicinal herbs.

The Mesopotamians believed that herbs had the power to cure a wide range of ailments, from minor injuries to serious diseases. They used herbs in a variety of ways, including in teas, potions, and ointments.

One of the most commonly used herbs in Mesopotamian medicine was the willow tree. The willow tree was used to treat fever, rheumatism and headaches to name a few. It was also used to treat wounds and to reduce inflammation.

Another important herb used in Mesopotamia was the opium poppy. The opium poppy was used to treat a variety of ailments, including pain, insomnia, and anxiety. It was also used as a sedative and as a treatment for a variety of mental health disorders.

Herbs used to treat respiratory problems

In ancient Mesopotamia, the region that is now modern-day Iraq, Kuwait, and parts of Syria, Turkey, and Iran, the people relied heavily on herbs to treat various ailments, including respiratory issues. The region's unique climate, with its hot summers and cold winters, made respiratory problems a common occurrence. The Mesopotamians developed a sophisticated understanding of herbal medicine, which they used to treat a range of respiratory conditions, from bronchitis and asthma to pneumonia and tuberculosis. Some of the most commonly used herbs for respiratory problems included:

Thyme (Thymus vulgaris): Known for its antibacterial and antiinflammatory properties, thyme was used to treat bronchitis, pneumonia, and other respiratory infections. It was believed to have antiinflammatory properties and was often used in combination with other herbs to treat respiratory problems.

Marjoram (Origanum majorana): A member of the mint family, marjoram was used to treat coughs, colds, and other respiratory infections. It was believed to have expectorant properties, helping to loosen and clear mucus from the lungs.

Lavender (Lavandula angustifolia): Lavender's calming properties made it a popular treatment for insomnia, anxiety, and stress-related respiratory problems, it was used to treat respiratory problems such as bronchitis and asthma. It was believed to have calming properties and was often used in combination with other herbs to treat anxiety and stress, which can exacerbate respiratory problems.

Eucalyptus (Eucalyptus globulus): Eucalyptus was used to treat respiratory problems such as bronchitis, pneumonia, and tuberculosis. It was believed to have decongestant and antiinflammatory properties, helping to relieve congestion and inflammation in the lungs.

Ginger (Zingiber officinale): Ginger was also used to treat respiratory problems such as bronchitis and asthma. It was believed to have antiinflammatory properties and was often used in combination with other herbs to treat digestive problems, which can be linked to respiratory issues.

Herbs used to treat digestive problems

In ancient Mesopotamia, digestive health was considered crucial for overall well-being. A healthy digestive system was seen as essential for maintaining good health and any disruptions to the digestive process were viewed as a serious concern. The Mesopotamians believed that the digestive system was closely linked to the body's overall health, and that any imbalance in the digestive system could lead to a range of health problems.

Digestive problems were also a common issue in ancient Mesopotamia, and the region's herbalists developed a range of remedies to treat them. Their knowledge of herbs was passed down through generations, and many of these remedies continue to be used today. Herbs such as cumin, thyme, and wormwood were used to treat digestive problems such as indigestion, diarrhea, and constipation. Some of the most commonly used herbs for digestive problems included:

Ginger (Zingiber officinale): Known for its anti-inflammatory properties, ginger was used to treat indigestion, nausea, and other digestive ailments. It was believed to have anti-inflammatory properties, which helped to reduce inflammation in the digestive tract and alleviate symptoms.

Fennel (Foeniculum vulgare): Fennel's carminative properties made it a popular treatment for bloating, gas, and other digestive issues.

Licorice root (Glycyrrhiza glabra): Licorice root's soothing properties made it a popular treatment for stomach ulcers, heartburn, and other digestive problems. Licorice was used to treat digestive issues such as indigestion, bloating, and diarrhea. *Myrrh* (Commiphora molmol): Myrrh was used to treat a range of digestive issues, including indigestion, bloating, and diarrhea.

Turmeric (Curcuma longa): Turmeric was used to treat digestive issues such as indigestion, bloating, and diarrhea.

Saffron (Crocus sativus): Saffron was also used to treat digestive issues such as indigestion, bloating, and diarrhea.

Herbs used to treat wounds, skin conditions, insect bites and stings

Herbs such as myrrh, cedar and thyme were used to treat wounds, skin condition, and other skin-related problems. Skin problems were a common issue in ancient Mesopotamia and the region's herbalists developed a range of remedies to treat them. Some of the most commonly used herbs for skin problems included:

Calendula (Calendula officinalis): Known for its anti-inflammatory and antibacterial properties, calendula was used to treat wounds, burns and other skin irritations. Calendula was used to treat skin conditions such as eczema and dermatitis. It was believed to have anti-inflammatory and soothing properties and was often used in combination with other herbs to treat skin conditions.

Aloe vera (Aloe barbadensis): Aloe vera's soothing properties made it a popular treatment for skin conditions such as eczema, acne and psoriasis. It was believed to have anti-inflammatory and soothing properties, and was often used in combination with other herbs to treat skin conditions.

Myrrh (Commiphora molmol): Myrrh's antiseptic properties

made it a popular treatment for wounds, cuts, and other skin irritations. Myrrh was used to treat a range of skin conditions, including eczema, acne, and skin infections. It was believed to have antiseptic and anti-inflammatory properties, and was often used in combination with other herbs to treat skin conditions.

Cedar: Cedar was used to treat skin conditions such as psoriasis and dermatitis. It was used to treat wounds and was believed to have antiseptic and anti-inflammatory properties.

Cypress: Cypress was used to treat skin conditions such as eczema and acne.

Chamomile: Chamomile was used to treat skin conditions such as eczema and dermatitis.

Lavender: Lavender was used to treat skin conditions such as acne and dermatitis. *Thyme:* Thyme was used to treat skin conditions such as eczema and dermatitis.

Licorice Root: Licorice root was used to treat skin conditions such as eczema and dermatitis.

Herbs used to treat mental health

Mental health was a significant concern in ancient Mesopotamia and the region's herbalists developed a range of remedies to treat mental health issues. Some of the most commonly used herbs for mental health included:

Ashwagandha (Withania somnifera): Known for its adaptogenic properties, ashwagandha was used to treat anxiety, stress, and other mental health issues.

Valerian (Valeriana officinalis): Valerian's sedative properties made it a popular treatment for insomnia, anxiety, and other mental health issues.

Lavender (Lavandula angustifolia): Lavender's calming properties made it a popular treatment for anxiety, stress, and other mental health issues.

The Legacy of Mesopotamian Herbalism in Modern Times

Despite the passage of thousands of years, the legacy of Mesopotamian herbalism
continues to influence the way we approach healthcare and wellness today.

Mesopotamian herbalism was a cornerstone of ancient Mesopotamian medicine, with a rich history dating back to the Sumerian civilization around 4500 BCE. The Mesopotamians believed that plants held the key to healing, and their understanding of botany and pharmacology was unparalleled in their time. They developed a sophisticated system of medicine that relied heavily on the use of herbs, which they believed could cure a wide range of ailments, from minor complaints to life-threatening diseases. One of the most significant contributions of Mesopotamian herbalism to modern medicine is the development of the concept of pharmacology. The Mesopotamians were among the first to recognize the importance of understanding the properties and actions of plants, and they developed a system of classification and categorization that allowed them to identify the most effective and safe herbal remedies. This approach to medicine laid the foundation for the development of modern pharmacology, which continues to play a crucial role in the treatment of diseases today. Many of the herbs used by the Mesopotamians are still used today, often in combination with modern pharmaceuticals, to treat a wide range of conditions. For example, the herb

myrrh, which was highly valued by the Mesopotamians for its antiseptic and anti-inflammatory properties, is still used today to treat wounds and infections. In addition, the concept of holistic medicine, which emphasizes the interconnectedness of the body and the importance of treating the whole person, rather than just the symptoms of a disease, is a key principle of Mesopotamian herbalism. This approach to medicine is gaining popularity in modern times, as people increasingly seek more natural and holistic approaches to healthcare.

The impact of Mesopotamian herbalism on modern medicine is far-reaching and multifaceted. The development of pharmacology, as mentioned earlier, is one of the most significant contributions of Mesopotamian herbalism to modern medicine. Additionally, the use of herbs in traditional medicine continues to influence the development of modern pharmaceuticals, with many modern medicines being derived from plants used by the Mesopotamians. Furthermore, the emphasis on holistic medicine and the importance of understanding the properties and actions of plants, which are key principles of Mesopotamian herbalism, continue to shape the way we approach healthcare today.

4

Herbs in Ancient Egypt

History of Herbs in Ancient Egypt

Ancient Egypt, a civilization that flourished along the Nile River, is renowned for its rich cultural heritage, architectural marvels, and sophisticated medical practices. Herbs played a vital role in the daily lives of the Egyptians, who utilized them for a wide range of purposes, from culinary and medicinal applications to spiritual and religious rituals. Ancient Egypt was renowned for its advanced understanding of herbal medicine, with a rich tradition of using plants to treat a wide range of ailments. The Egyptians believed that the gods had given them the gift of healing, and they spent centuries developing a sophisticated system of medicine that relied heavily on the use of herbs.

Medicinal Uses

The Egyptians were skilled in the art of medicine, and herbs played a crucial role in their healing practices. They used herbs to treat a wide range of ailments, from fever and rheumatism to skin conditions and digestive issues. The Egyptians believed that herbs possessed magical properties, and many were used in combination with other substances to create potent remedies. For example, the herb *chamomile* was used to treat anxiety and insomnia, while the herb sage was used to treat digestive issues. The Egyptians also used herbs to create ointments, salves, and poultices to treat wounds and skin conditions.

Ancient Egypt was renowned for its advanced understanding and utilization of medicinal herbs. The Egyptians believed in the concept of "ma'at," which referred to the balance and harmony of the universe, and they applied this principle to their approach to medicine. They recognized the importance of maintaining balance in the body and used herbs to achieve this balance.

One of the most commonly used herbs in Ancient Egyptian medicine was the *papyrus plant.* The Egyptians believed that papyrus had a number of healing properties, including the ability to reduce inflammation and ease pain. It was often used to treat conditions such as arthritis and gout, and was also used to create a type of ointment that was applied to the skin to soothe and calm irritated areas.

Another important herb used by the Egyptians was the *willow tree.* The bark of the willow tree contains salicylic acid, a compound that is similar to aspirin and has anti-inflammatory properties. The Egyptians used the bark of the willow tree to create a type of medicine that was used to treat headaches, fever, and other conditions.

The Egyptians also used a variety of herbs to treat digestive problems. For example, they used the leaves of the *coriander* plant to treat indigestion and other stomach ailments. The seeds of the coriander plant were also used to treat a variety of conditions, including respiratory problems and skin irritations.

The use of herbs in Ancient Egyptian medicine was not limited to treating physical conditions. The Egyptians also used herbs to treat mental and emotional conditions, such as anxiety and depression. For example, they used the leaves of the chamomile plant to create a type of tea that was believed to have a calming effect on the mind and body.

Herbs Used in Ancient Egyptian Medicine

The Egyptians used a wide range of herbs to treat various ailments, including digestive issues, skin problems, and respiratory infections. Some of the most commonly used herbs include:

Calendula (Calendula officinalis): This herb was used to treat skin conditions such as eczema, acne, and wounds. It was also used to soothe burns and reduce inflammation.

Chamomile (Matricaria chamomilla): Chamomile was used to treat digestive issues such as indigestion, nausea, and insomnia. It was also used to calm anxiety and promote relaxation.

Dill (Anethum graveolens): Dill was used to treat digestive issues such as indigestion, bloating, and gas. It was also used to reduce fever and alleviate symptoms of the common cold.

Fennel (Foeniculum vulgare): Fennel was used to treat digestive issues such as indigestion, bloating, and gas. It was also used to reduce fever and alleviate symptoms of the common cold.

Garlic (Allium sativum): Garlic was used to treat a variety of ailments, including respiratory infections, digestive issues, and skin problems. It was also used to repel insects and improve circulation.

Ginger (Zingiber officinale): Ginger was used to treat digestive issues such as nausea, indigestion, and bloating. It was also used to reduce inflammation and alleviate symptoms of the common cold.

Lavender (Lavandula angustifolia): Lavender was used to treat anxiety, insomnia, and skin conditions such as acne and eczema. It was also used to promote relaxation and reduce stress.

Marjoram (Origanum majorana): Marjoram was used to treat digestive issues such as indigestion, bloating, and gas. It was also used to reduce fever and alleviate symptoms of the common cold.

Mint (Mentha piperita): Mint was used to treat digestive issues such as indigestion, bloating, and gas. It was also used to reduce fever and alleviate symptoms of the common cold.

Sage (Salvia officinalis): Sage was used to treat digestive issues such as indigestion, bloating, and gas. It was also used to reduce fever and alleviate symptoms of the common cold.

Saffron, which was used to treat fever and rheumatism

Myrrh, which was used to treat skin diseases and wounds

Galen, which was used to treat mental health conditions

Applications of Medicinal Herbs in Ancient Egyptian Medicine

The Egyptians used medicinal herbs in a variety of ways, including:

Infusions: Herbs were steeped in hot water to create a tea-like concoction that was used to treat various ailments.

Decoctions: Herbs were boiled in water to create a strong liquid extract that was used to treat more severe conditions.

Poultices: Herbs were applied topically to the skin to treat skin conditions such as wounds, burns, and eczema.

Inhalations: Herbs were inhaled to treat respiratory infections such as bronchitis and asthma.

Enemas: Herbs were used to treat digestive issues such as constipation and diarrhea.

Suppositories: Herbs were used to treat vaginal infections and other genital issues.

Capsules: Herbs were used to treat digestive issues such as indigestion and bloating.

The Egyptians also used medicinal herbs in combination with other treatments, such as surgery, massage, and meditation. They believed that the key to successful treatment lay in understanding the underlying causes of the ailment and using a combination of treatments to restore balance to the body.

The use of herbs in Ancient Egyptian medicine is a testament to the ingenuity and resourcefulness of the ancient Egyptians, and provides a fascinating glimpse into the ways in which they used plants to promote health and well-being.

Internal Ailments - Diseases

One of the most common internal ailments treated with herbs in ancient Egypt was *digestive issues*. The Egyptians believed that a healthy digestive system was essential for overall well-being, and they used a variety of herbs to treat conditions such as indigestion, constipation, and diarrhea. For example, they used the herb *chamomile* to soothe digestive issues, while the herb *coriander* was used to treat indigestion and bloating. The Egyptians also used the herb *fennel* to treat digestive issues, as it was believed to have a calming effect on the stomach.

Another common internal ailment treated with herbs in ancient Egypt was *respiratory issues*. The Egyptians believed that the lungs were responsible for the body's vital energy, and they used a variety of herbs to treat conditions such as bronchitis, asthma, and pneumonia. For example, they used the herb *thyme* to treat respiratory issues, as it was believed to have antibacterial properties. The Egyptians also used the herb *eucalyptus* to treat respiratory issues, as it was believed to have a decongestant effect. In addition to digestive and respiratory issues, the Egyptians also used herbs to treat a range of other internal ailments, including fever, rheumatism, and skin conditions. For example, they used the herb *willow bark* to treat fever, as it was believed to have anti-inflammatory properties. The Egyptians also used the herb *lavender* to treat skin conditions, as it was believed to have
antiseptic properties.

The Egyptians also used herbs to treat a range of mental and emotional disorders, including anxiety, depression, and insomnia. For example, they used the herb valerian root to treat insomnia, as it was believed to have a sedative effect. The

Egyptians also used the herb chamomile to treat anxiety and depression for its calming effect on the mind and body.

One of the most significant contributions of Ancient Egyptian medicine was the use of herbal remedies. The Egyptians believed that plants had healing properties and used them to treat a wide range of ailments. They believed that the gods had given them the gift of healing and that they could use this gift to cure diseases.

The Egyptians used herbs to treat various conditions, including fever, rheumatism, and skin diseases. They also used herbs to treat mental health conditions, such as anxiety and depression. The Egyptians believed that the use of herbs could help to balance the body's humors, which they believed were responsible for maintaining good health.

The Egyptians also used herbs to treat various types of injuries, including wounds and burns. They believed that the use of herbs could help to promote healing and prevent infection.

Herbal Remedies in Medical Texts

The ancient Egyptians were renowned for their extensive knowledge of herbal remedies, which played a significant role in their medical practices. The use of herbs in medicine was deeply rooted in their culture and was often mentioned in various medical texts.

The Edwin Smith Papyrus, one of the most significant medical texts from ancient Egypt, dates back to around 1600 BCE. This papyrus is a collection of medical cases and treatments, including the use of herbal remedies. The text describes the use of herbs such as chamomile, coriander, and myrrh to treat various conditions, including wounds, fever, and digestive issues. For instance, the papyrus recommends applying a mixture of chamomile and coriander to wounds to promote healing and prevent infection.

The Ebers Papyrus, another important medical text from ancient Egypt, dates back to around 1550 BCE. This papyrus is a comprehensive medical text that covers a wide range of topics, including the use of herbal remedies. The text describes the use of herbs such as opium, mandrake, and henbane to treat various conditions, including pain, insomnia, and mental disorders. For example, the papyrus recommends using opium to treat pain and reduce Inflammation.

The papyrus of Hearst, which dates back to around 1500 BCE, describes the use of herbs such as lavender and valerian to treat anxiety and insomnia. The text also recommends using herbs such as mandrake and henbane to treat mental disorders, including depression and hysteria.

The use of herbal remedies in ancient Egyptian medicine was not limited to the treatment of specific ailments. The Egyptians also used herbs to promote overall health and well-being. The papyrus of Hearst, for example, describes the use of herbs such as chamomile and coriander to promote digestion and relieve stress. The text also recommends using herbs such as lavender and valerian to promote relaxation and reduce anxiety.

5

Greece

History of Herbal Medicine in Ancient Greece

Ancient Greece was a civilization that thrived from around 8th century BCE to 146 CE, leaving behind a rich legacy of art, architecture, philosophy, and medicine. The ancient Greeks were known for their contributions to the field of medicine, which was deeply rooted in the use of herbs and other natural substances.

Early Beginnings

The use of herbs in ancient Greece dates back to the earliest times, with evidence of herbal remedies found in the Linear B tablets of the Mycenaean civilization (16th-12th centuries BCE). The tablets contain references to various herbs, including *saffron, thyme* and *coriander*, which were used for both medicinal and culinary purposes. The use of herbs was also mentioned in the works of Homer, the ancient Greek poet, who wrote about the healing properties of plants in his epic poems, the Iliad and the Odyssey.

The Role of Herbs in Ancient Greek Medicine

In ancient Greek medicine, herbs played a crucial role in the treatment of various ailments. The Greek physician Hippocrates (460-370 BCE), known as the father of medicine, emphasized the importance of using natural substances, including herbs, in the treatment of diseases. Hippocrates believed that the body had the ability to heal itself, and that the role of the physician was to assist this process by using natural remedies.

The Greek physician Galen (129-216 CE) also relied heavily on herbs in his medical practice. Galen believed that the body was composed of four humors (blood, phlegm, yellow bile, and black bile), and that an imbalance of these humors could lead to disease. He used herbs to balance the humors and restore health to the body.

Commonly Used Herbs

Many herbs were used in ancient Greek medicine, including:

Saffron (Crocus sativus): used to treat a variety of ailments, including insomnia, digestive problems, and skin conditions.

Thyme (Thymus vulgaris): used to treat respiratory problems, such as coughs and bronchitis.

Coriander (Coriandrum sativum): used to treat digestive problems, such as indigestion and diarrhea.

Mint (Mentha piperita): used to treat digestive problems, such as indigestion and nausea.

Sage (Salvia officinalis): used to treat memory loss and

cognitive impairment.

Lavender (Lavandula angustifolia): used to treat anxiety and insomnia.

Herbal Remedies

Ancient Greek physicians used a variety of herbal remedies, including:

Infusions: a mixture of herbs steeped in water or wine.

Decoctions: a mixture of herbs boiled in water or wine.

Poultices: a mixture of herbs applied topically to the skin.

Salves: a mixture of herbs and oils applied topically to the skin.

Tinctures: a mixture of herbs and water or wine taken orally.

Respiratory Issues & Herbs for Coughs

In Ancient Greece, respiratory issues were a common affliction, particularly during the harsh winters and humid summers. The Greeks relied heavily on traditional herbal medicine to alleviate symptoms and promote overall health.

Thyme (Thymus vulgaris): Thyme was a staple in Greek medicine, used to treat a variety of respiratory issues, including coughs. The essential oils present in thyme, such as thymol, possess antibacterial and anti-inflammatory properties, making it an effective natural remedy for coughs.

Lemon Balm (Melissa officinalis): Lemon balm, a member of the mint family, was used to calm coughs and soothe the throat. Its mild, citrusy flavor made it a popular ingredient in teas and infusions.

Elderflower (Sambucus nigra): Elderflower was used to

treat a range of respiratory issues, including coughs, colds, and bronchitis. Its antiviral and anti-inflammatory properties helped to reduce inflammation and ease congestion.

Honey and Sage (Salvia officinalis): Honey was a common ingredient in Greek medicine, often used to soothe coughs and calm the throat. Sage, with its natural antibacterial properties, was added to honey to create a potent cough syrup.

Herbs for Colds

Colds were a common occurrence in Ancient Greece, often caused by viral infections or exposure to cold temperatures. The Greeks employed a range of herbs to alleviate symptoms and promote recovery. Some of the most commonly used herbs for colds include:

Echinacea (Echinacea spp.): Echinacea was used to boost the immune system and reduce the severity of cold symptoms. Its antiinflammatory and antiviral properties helped to alleviate congestion and reduce the risk of complications.

Ginger (Zingiber officinale): Ginger was used to treat a range of respiratory issues, including colds, coughs, and bronchitis. Its natural anti-inflammatory properties helped to reduce inflammation and ease congestion.

Eucalyptus (Eucalyptus globulus): Eucalyptus was used to treat respiratory issues, including colds, coughs, and bronchitis. Its essential oils, such as eucalyptol, possess decongestant and anti-inflammatory properties, making it an effective natural remedy for colds.

Yarrow (Achillea millefolium): Yarrow was used to treat a range of respiratory issues, including colds, coughs, and bronchitis. Its antiseptic and anti-inflammatory properties helped to reduce inflammation and promote recovery.

Herbs for Bronchitis and Asthma

Bronchitis and asthma were common respiratory issues in Ancient Greece, often caused by environmental factors, allergies, or respiratory infections. The Greeks employed a range of herbs to alleviate symptoms and promote recovery. Some of the most commonly used herbs for bronchitis and asthma include:

Marshmallow (Althaea officinalis): Marshmallow was used to soothe and calm irritated airways, reducing inflammation and congestion. Its mucilages helped to protect the mucous membranes and promote healing.

Licorice (Glycyrrhiza glabra): Licorice was used to treat a range of respiratory issues, including bronchitis, asthma, and coughs. Its antiinflammatory properties helped to reduce inflammation and ease congestion.

Elecampane (Inula helenium): Elecampane was used to treat respiratory issues, including bronchitis, asthma, and coughs. Its antiseptic and anti-inflammatory properties helped to reduce inflammation and promote recovery.

Borage (Borago officinalis): Borage was used to treat respiratory issues, including bronchitis, asthma, and coughs. Its essential oils, such as borage oil, possess anti-inflammatory properties, making it an effective natural remedy for respiratory issues.

Skin and Wound Care: Herbs used to treat skin conditions and wounds

In ancient Greece, herbal medicine played a significant role in the treatment of various skin conditions and wounds. The Greeks recognized the importance of using natural remedies to promote healing, prevent infection and alleviate symptoms.

Calendula (Calendula officinalis): Known as "golden petals," calendula was used to treat a range of skin conditions, including acne, eczema, and dermatitis. The flowers were infused in oil or water to create a soothing topical application.

Lavender (Lavandula angustifolia): Lavender was used to calm irritated skin, reduce inflammation, and promote relaxation. The essential oil was often added to bathwater or used as a compress to soothe skin irritations.

Marigold (Calendula officinalis): Marigold was used to treat skin conditions such as eczema, acne, and rosacea. The flowers were infused in oil or water to create a topical application that reduced inflammation and promoted healing.

Plantain (Plantago major): Plantain was used to treat skin irritations, wounds, and burns. The leaves were crushed and applied topically to reduce inflammation and promote healing.

Witch Hazel (Hamamelis virginiana): Witch hazel was used to treat wounds, cuts, and abrasions. The bark was infused in water to create a topical application that reduced inflammation, promoted healing, and prevented infection.

Comfrey (Symphytum officinale): Comfrey was used to treat wounds, burns, and ulcers. The leaves were crushed and applied topically to promote healing, reduce inflammation, and prevent infection.

Yarrow (Achillea millefolium): Yarrow was used to treat

wounds, cuts, and abrasions. The leaves were crushed and applied topically to promote healing, reduce inflammation, and prevent infection.

Garlic (Allium sativum): Garlic was used to treat wounds, cuts, and abrasions. The crushed cloves were applied topically to promote healing, reduce inflammation, and prevent infection.

Digestive Health: Herbs used to treat digestive issues and promote overall health

In ancient Greece, traditional herbal medicine played a significant role in the treatment of various health conditions, including digestive issues. The Greeks recognized the importance of maintaining a healthy digestive system, which they believed was closely linked to overall well-being.

Dittany of Crete (Origanum dictamnus): This herb was used to treat a range of digestive problems, including indigestion, bloating, and abdominal pain. It was believed to have anti-inflammatory properties and was often used in combination with other herbs to treat digestive issues.

Fennel (Foeniculum vulgare): Fennel was used to treat digestive problems such as indigestion, bloating, and flatulence. It was believed to have carminative properties, which helped to relieve gas and bloating.

Ginger (Zingiber officinale): Ginger was used to treat a range of digestive problems, including nausea, vomiting, and indigestion. It was believed to have anti-inflammatory properties and was often used in combination with other herbs to treat digestive issues.

Licorice root (Glycyrrhiza glabra): Licorice root was used to treat digestive problems such as stomach ulcers, heartburn, and indigestion. It was believed to have anti-inflammatory properties and was often used in combination with other herbs to treat digestive issues.

Marjoram (Origanum majorana), **Peppermint** (Mentha piperita), **Sage** (Salvia officinalis) and **Thyme** (Thymus vulgaris) was used to treat digestive problems such as indigestion, bloating, and abdominal pain.

Influence on Later Medicine

The use of herbs in ancient Greek medicine had a lasting impact on the development of medicine in later centuries. The Greek physician Dioscorides (40-90 CE) wrote a comprehensive book on herbal medicine, De Materia Medica, which became a standard reference for physicians for centuries. The use of herbs continued to evolve over time, with the development of new remedies and the discovery of new herbs.

Galen and the Development of Herbal Medicine

Galen (129-216 CE) was a Greek physician who was heavily influenced by the teachings of Hippocrates. Galen was a prolific writer who wrote extensively on a range of medical topics, including the use of herbal medicine. Galen believed that the body was made up of four fluid-like substances, known as "humors," which needed to be balanced in order to maintain health. He developed a range of herbal remedies that were designed to balance the humors and promote health.

Galen was particularly interested in the use of herbs to treat mental health conditions, such as anxiety and depression. He believed that the use of herbs could help to balance the humors and promote a sense of well-being. Galen developed a range of herbal remedies that were designed to treat mental health conditions, including the use of herbs such as *lavender* and *chamomile*.

Galen's work on herbal medicine was highly influential, and his writings on the subject were widely read and studied for centuries. His emphasis on the importance of balancing the humors and using herbal remedies to promote health and well-being had a lasting impact on the development of traditional herbal medicine.

The Legacy of Hippocrates and Galen

The contributions of Hippocrates and Galen to the development of herbal medicine are still felt today. Their emphasis on the importance of observation, experimentation, and the use of natural remedies has had a lasting impact on the practice of traditional medicine. The use of herbal remedies to promote health and well-being is still a popular practice today, and the work of Hippocrates and Galen continues to influence the development of new herbal remedies.

6

Traditional Chinese Medicine

History of Traditional Chinese Medicine: Overview of the Origins and Development of Traditional Chinese Medicine

Traditional Chinese Medicine (TCM) has a rich and complex history that spans over 2,500 years. It has evolved from a combination of ancient Chinese philosophy, mythology, and medical practices to become a distinct system of medicine that is still widely used today.

TCM herbs are derived from plants, animals, and minerals, and are used to restore balance to the body's energy, or "qi." In TCM, the body is seen as a complex system of interconnected organs and pathways, and the use of herbs is based on the principle of treating the whole person, rather than just the symptoms of a disease. TCM herbs are often used in combination with other TCM therapies, such as acupuncture and massage, to promote health and well-being.

32

Early Beginnings: The Roots of Traditional Chinese Medicine

The earliest recorded evidence of traditional Chinese medicine dates back to the Shang Dynasty (16th-11th centuries BCE). During this period, Chinese medicine was heavily influenced by the concept of yin and yang, the five elements, and the theory of qi. These fundamental principles would later become the foundation of TCM.

The Huangdi Neijing (Yellow Emperor's Inner Canon), a foundational text of TCM, is believed to have been written during the Han Dynasty (206 BCE-220 CE). This text describes the concept of qi, the flow of energy in the body, and the importance of maintaining balance and harmony.

The Golden Age of Traditional Chinese Medicine

The Tang Dynasty (618-907 CE) is often referred to as the "Golden Age" of TCM. During this period, Chinese medicine experienced a significant surge in development, with the establishment of the Imperial Medical Academy and the creation of the first comprehensive medical textbook, the "Ben Cao Gang Mu" (Compendium of Materia Medica).

The Tang Dynasty also saw the rise of famous Chinese physicians, such as Li Shizhen, who wrote the "Ben Cao Gang Mu" and made significant contributions to the field of pharmacology. His work remains a cornerstone of TCM to this day.

Influence of Buddhism and Taoism

Buddhism and Taoism had a profound impact on the development of TCM. Buddhist concepts such as karma, reincarnation, and the importance of spiritual practices influenced the development of TCM's philosophical framework. Taoist principles, such as the concept of wu wei (non-action) and the importance of living in harmony with nature, also shaped TCM's approach to health and medicine. The Taoist emphasis on the interconnectedness of all things and the balance between yin and yang is reflected in TCM's emphasis on maintaining balance and harmony in the body.

Modern Developments and Challenges

In the 20th century, TCM faced significant challenges, including the rise of Western medicine and the Cultural Revolution. However, TCM continued to evolve, with the establishment of the China Academy of Traditional Chinese Medicine in 1954 and the development of new techniques, such as acupuncture and moxibustion.

Today, TCM is recognized as a distinct system of medicine, with its own unique theories, practices, and philosophies. It is practiced not only in China but also around the world, with many countries incorporating TCM into their healthcare systems.

The Concept of Herbology

Herbology is the study of the use of herbs in TCM. Herbs are used to tonify, sedate, warm, cool, and move the body's energies and to treat a wide range of conditions. Herbs can be used in various forms, including raw, cooked, decocted, or combined with other herbs.

The Concept of Formulae

Formulae are combinations of herbs that are used to treat specific patterns and conditions. Formulae can be tailored to an individual's unique needs and can be used to treat a wide range of conditions, from common colds to chronic diseases.

The Concept of Meridian Theory

Meridian theory is the study of the flow of Qi and blood through the body. Practitioners use meridian theory to diagnose and treat imbalances and blockages in the flow of Qi and blood.

Types of Herbs: Classification and Characteristics of Different Types of Herbs Used in TCM

Traditional Chinese Medicine (TCM) has a rich history of utilizing herbs to treat various health conditions. The use of herbs in TCM dates back thousands of years, with records of herbal remedies found in ancient Chinese texts such as the Shennong Ben Cao Jing and the Ben Cao Gang Mu. In TCM, herbs are classified into different categories based on their characteristics, functions, and properties.

Classification of Herbs in TCM

Herbs in TCM are classified into three main categories: roots, stems, and leaves. Each category is further sub-classified into different types based on their properties, functions, and characteristics.

Roots

Roots are the most commonly used herbs in TCM. They are typically harvested from plants that have a strong, concentrated energy. Roots are often used to treat conditions related to the kidneys, liver, and spleen. Some common types of root herbs include:

Ginseng (Ren Shen): Known for its adaptogenic properties, ginseng is used to tonify the Qi and improve overall health.

Astragalus (Huang Qi): Astragalus is used to tonify the Qi and boost the immune system.

Licorice root (Glycyrrhizae): Licorice root is used to harmonize the effects of other herbs and treat digestive disorders.

Stems

Stems are typically harvested from the middle or upper part of the plant. They are often used to treat conditions related to the heart, liver, and spleen. Some common types of stem herbs include:

Dong quai (Angelica sinensis): Dong quai is used to tonify the blood and treat menstrual disorders.

Schisandra (Wu Wei Zi): Schisandra is used to tonify the Qi and treat digestive disorders.

Gentiana (Long Dan Cao): Gentiana is used to clear heat and treat digestive disorders.

Leaves

Leaves are typically harvested from the upper part of the plant. They are often used to treat conditions related to the lungs, liver, and kidneys. Some common types of leaf herbs include:

Peppermint (Bo He): Peppermint is used to clear heat and treat digestive disorders.

Lemon balm (Mentha citrata): Lemon balm is used to calm the spirit and treat anxiety.

Chrysanthemum (Ju Hua): Chrysanthemum is used to clear heat and treat respiratory disorders.

Other Types of Herbs

In addition to roots, stems, and leaves, TCM also uses other types of herbs,

Flowers: Flowers are used to treat conditions related to the heart, liver, and kidneys. Examples include *rose petals* (Jiaozhi) and *jasmine flowers* (Mai Hua).

Fruits: Fruits are used to treat conditions related to the liver, kidneys, and digestive system. Examples include *Chinese dates* (Zi Zhi) and *Chinese angelica* (Dong Quai).

Seeds: Seeds are used to treat conditions related to the liver, kidneys, and digestive system. Examples include *sesame seeds* (Hei Zhi) and *Chinese angelica seeds* (Dong Quai Zi).

Bark: Bark is used to treat conditions related to the liver, kidneys, and digestive system. Examples include *cinnamon bark* (Rou Gui) and *magnolia bark* (Hou Po).

Resin: Resin is used to treat conditions related to the liver, kidneys, and digestive system. Examples include *frankincense resin* (Ru Xiang) and *myrrh resin* (Mo Yao).

Properties and Functions of Herbs

Herbs in TCM are classified into different properties and functions based on their characteristics. The properties of herbs include:

Cold: Herbs that are cold in nature are used to treat conditions related to heat and inflammation. Examples include *peppermint* (Bo He) and *chrysanthemum* (Ju Hua).

Hot: Herbs that are hot in nature are used to treat conditions related to cold and stagnation. Examples include *ginger* (Gan Cao) and *cinnamon* (Rou Gui).

Warm: Herbs that are warm in nature are used to treat conditions related to cold and stagnation. Examples include *ginger* (Gan Cao) and *clove* (Ding Xiang).

Cool: Herbs that are cool in nature are used to treat conditions related to heat and inflammation. Examples include *mint* (Bo He) and *chrysanthemum* (Ju Hua).

The functions of herbs include:

Tonifying: Herbs that tonify are used to strengthen and nourish the body. Examples include *ginseng* (Ren Shen) and *astragalus* (Huang Qi).

Sedating: Herbs that sedate are used to calm the spirit and treat anxiety. Examples include *lemon balm* (Mentha citrata) and *valerian* (Jie Geng).

Invigorating: Herbs that invigorate are used to stimulate the body and treat fatigue. Examples include *ginseng* (Ren Shen) and *licorice root* (Glycyrrhizae).

Clearing: Herbs that clear are used to remove heat and toxins from the body. Examples include *chrysanthemum* (Ju Hua) and *dandelion* (Pu Gong Ying).

Herbal Formulations: Combining Herbs to Create Effective Remedies for Various Health Conditions

In traditional Chinese medicine, herbal formulations play a crucial role in treating a wide range of health conditions. By combining different herbs, practitioners can create unique blends that address specific patterns of disharmony in the body.

Principles of Herbal Formulation

Before delving into specific examples of herbal formulations, it's essential to understand the underlying principles that guide their creation. In traditional Chinese medicine, herbal formulations are designed to address specific patterns of disharmony, known as "patterns of disease." These patterns are determined by a combination of factors, including the individual's constitutional type, environmental factors, and lifestyle choices. The principles of herbal formulation in traditional Chinese medicine can be summarized as follows:

Synergy: The whole is greater than the sum of its parts. Each herb in a formulation works together to create a synergistic effect that is greater than the individual herbs alone.

Balance: Herbal formulations aim to restore balance to the body by addressing specific patterns of disharmony. This is achieved by combining herbs that have complementary properties and actions.

Specificity: Each herbal formulation is designed to address a specific pattern of disease or health condition. Practitioners must carefully select herbs that are tailored to the individual's unique needs.

Gradation: Herbal formulations are designed to be graduated, meaning that the strength and potency of the herbs can be adjusted to suit the individual's needs.

Techniques for Creating Herbal Formulations

There are several techniques that practitioners use to create effective herbal formulations. These include:

Layering: This involves combining herbs that have different properties and actions to create a layered effect. For example, a practitioner might combine a warming herb with a cooling herb to create a balanced formula.

Blending: This involves combining herbs that have similar properties and actions to create a harmonious blend. For example, a practitioner might combine three herbs that have similar warming properties to create a formula that is both warming and harmonious.

Contrasting: This involves combining herbs that have opposite properties and actions to create a contrasting effect. For example, a practitioner might combine a warming herb with a cooling herb to create a formula that is both warming and cooling.

Examples of Herbal Formulations

Four Winds Formula: This formula is used to treat respiratory conditions such as bronchitis and asthma. It combines four herbs: *ginseng, licorice root, apricot kernel, and ephedra.*

Eight Treasures Formula: This formula is used to treat digestive conditions such as constipation and diarrhea. It combines eight herbs: *ginseng, licorice root, apricot kernel, ephedra, magnolia bark, citrus peel, and ginger.*

Three Yin Formula: This formula is used to treat menstrual cramps and other gynecological conditions. It combines three herbs: *angelica root, cinnamon bark, and licorice root.*

Formulations and Preparation Methods

In traditional Chinese medicine, herbal remedies are often prepared in the form of teas, soups, or capsules. The specific preparation method and dosage will depend on the individual's symptoms and health status. Some common formulations and preparation methods include:

Teas: Herbal teas are a popular way to prepare and consume herbal remedies. The herbs are typically steeped in hot water for a period of time, and then strained and consumed as a warm beverage.

Soups: Herbal soups are a nourishing and comforting way to consume herbal remedies. The herbs are typically simmered in water for a period of time, and then consumed as a warm soup.

Capsules: Herbal capsules are a convenient way to consume herbal remedies. The herbs are typically dried and powdered, and then filled into capsules that can be taken orally.

Herbs Used:

Ginseng

Ginseng is one of the most revered and widely used herbs in traditional Chinese medicine (TCM). Its unique properties and benefits have been recognized for centuries, and it is often referred to as the "king of herbs."

History and Classification

Ginseng has been used in traditional Chinese medicine for over 2,000 years, with records of its use dating back to the Han Dynasty (206 BCE - 220 CE). It is believed to have originated in the mountains of China, where it was highly prized for its medicinal properties. Today, ginseng is classified into several species, including Asian ginseng (Panax ginseng), American ginseng (Panax quinquefolius), and Siberian ginseng (Eleutherococcus senticosus).

Properties

Ginseng is known for its adaptogenic properties, which enable it to balance and regulate the body's physiological processes. It is believed to have the following properties:

Qi-tonifying: Ginseng is said to tonify (strengthen) the body's Qi, or vital energy, which is essential for maintaining overall health and well-being.

Yin-tonifying: Ginseng is also believed to tonify the body's Yin energy, which is responsible for cooling and moistening the body.

Blood-tonifying: Ginseng is said to tonify the body's blood, which is essential for maintaining healthy circulation and preventing blood related disorders.

Calming: Ginseng is believed to have a calming effect on the body, which can help to reduce stress and anxiety.

Uses

Decoction: Ginseng is often decocted in water to create a tea-like infusion that is consumed orally.

Capsules: Ginseng is also available in capsule form, which can be taken orally.

Topical application: Ginseng can be applied topically to the skin to treat various conditions, such as skin ulcers and wounds.

Benefits

Ginseng is believed to have numerous benefits in TCM, including:

Improving mental clarity and focus: Ginseng is said to improve mental clarity and focus by tonifying the brain and nervous system.

Enhancing physical performance: Ginseng is believed to enhance physical performance by increasing energy levels and improving endurance.

Reducing stress and anxiety: Ginseng is said to reduce stress and anxiety by calming the body and mind.

Improving sleep: Ginseng is believed to improve sleep quality by regulating the body's sleep-wake cycle.

Boosting immune function: Ginseng is said to boost immune function by tonifying the body's immune system.

Clinical Applications:

Ginseng is used to treat a variety of conditions in TCM, including:

Fatigue and weakness: Ginseng is often used to treat fatigue and weakness, particularly in individuals who are experiencing stress or burnout.

Insomnia: Ginseng is believed to improve sleep quality and is often used to treat insomnia.

Anxiety and depression: Ginseng is said to reduce stress and anxiety.

Digestive disorders: Ginseng is believed to have anti-inflammatory properties and is often used to treat digestive disorders, such as gastritis and colitis.

Cardiovascular disease: Ginseng is said to have cardiovascular protective effects and is often used to treat cardiovascular disease.

Astragalus

In traditional Chinese medicine (TCM), astragalus (Astragalus membranaceus) is a highly valued herb that has been used for centuries to promote health and prevent disease. Also known as Huang Qi, astragalus is a type of legume that is native to China and is widely cultivated for its medicinal properties.

Astragalus has been used in traditional Chinese medicine for over 2,000 years, dating back to the Han Dynasty (206 BCE - 220 CE). It was first mentioned in the famous Chinese medical text, the "Shennong Ben Cao Jing," which is considered one of the most important works on traditional Chinese medicine. Astragalus was highly valued for its ability to tonify the Qi, or vital energy, and was often used to treat a range of conditions, including respiratory problems, digestive issues, and fatigue. In TCM, astragalus is considered a "Qi-tonifying" herb, meaning that it is believed to help restore and balance the body's vital energy. It is often used in combination with other herbs to treat a variety of conditions, including:

Respiratory problems, such as bronchitis and pneumonia
Digestive issues, such as diarrhea and constipation
Fatigue and weakness
Immune system disorders, such as HIV and AIDS
Cancer and cancer treatment side effects

Properties

Astragalus is believed to have a number of properties that make it useful in TCM.

Qi-tonifying: Astragalus is believed to help restore and balance the body's vital energy, or Qi.

Anti-inflammatory: Astragalus has been shown to have antiinflammatory properties, which may help reduce swelling and pain.

Antioxidant: Astragalus contains antioxidants, which help protect the body from damage caused by free radicals.

Immune-modulating: Astragalus is believed to have immune-modulating properties, which may help regulate the immune system and prevent disease.

Preparation and Administration

Astragalus is typically prepared as a decoction, which involves boiling the herb in water to release its active compounds. The decoction is then strained and taken as a tea. Astragalus can also be taken in capsule or tablet form, or as a powder that is mixed with water or other liquids.

Licorice Root

Licorice root, also known as Gan Cao in Chinese, is one of the most widely used and revered herbs in traditional Chinese medicine (TCM). It has been used for thousands of years to treat a variety of health conditions, from digestive issues to respiratory problems.

Properties of Licorice Root

Licorice root is a sweet and slightly bitter herb that is rich in flavonoids, saponins, and glycyrrhizin. These compounds give licorice root its unique properties, which include:

Sweetness: Licorice root is known for its sweet taste, which makes it a popular ingredient in traditional Chinese medicine.

Anti-inflammatory properties: The flavonoids and saponins in licorice root have anti-inflammatory properties, which help to reduce swelling and pain.

Antiviral properties: Licorice root has been shown to have antiviral properties, which help to prevent the spread of viruses.

Soothing properties: Licorice root is often used to soothe digestive issues, such as heartburn and indigestion.

Uses of Licorice Root in TCM

Tea: Licorice root is often used to make a tea that can be consumed on its own or combined with other herbs.

Powder: Licorice root can be dried and powdered, which can be used to make capsules or added to other herbal remedies.

Tincture: Licorice root can be extracted into a tincture, which can be taken sublingually or added to other herbal remedies.

Cooking: Licorice root can be used in cooking, particularly in traditional Chinese dishes such as stir-fries and soups.

Benefits of Licorice Root in TCM

Digestive issues: Licorice root is often used to treat digestive issues such as heartburn, indigestion, and diarrhea.

Respiratory issues: Licorice root has been shown to be effective in treating respiratory issues such as bronchitis, asthma, and coughs.

Skin issues: Licorice root has anti-inflammatory properties, which can help to soothe skin issues such as acne, eczema, and psoriasis.

Stress and anxiety: Licorice root has been shown to have a calming effect on the nervous system, which can help to reduce stress and anxiety.

Traditional Chinese Medicine Applications of Licorice Root

Formulae: Licorice root is often used in combination with other herbs to create formulae that can be used to treat a variety of health conditions.

Tonification: Licorice root is often used to tonify the body, which means to nourish and strengthen the body's energy.

Sedation: Licorice root has a sedative effect, which can help to calm the body and mind.

Modern Applications of Licorice Root

Herbal medicine: Licorice root is used in herbal medicine to treat a variety of health conditions, from digestive issues to respiratory problems.

Cosmetics: Licorice root is used in cosmetics to soothe and calm the skin.

Food: Licorice root is used as a flavoring agent in food, particularly in Asian cuisine.

Cold and Flu: Herbal Remedies for Preventing and Treating Cold and Flu

In traditional Chinese medicine, the prevention and treatment of cold and flu are considered crucial for maintaining overall health and well-being. The use of herbs plays a significant role in this approach, as they offer a natural and effective way to boost the immune system, alleviate symptoms, and promote recovery. In this chapter, we will explore the various herbal remedies used in traditional Chinese medicine to prevent and treat cold and flu.

In traditional Chinese medicine, cold and flu are considered to be caused by an imbalance of the body's Qi, or life energy. This imbalance can occur when the body's defenses are weakened, allowing external pathogens, such as wind, cold, and dampness, to invade the body. The symptoms of cold and flu, such as fever, cough, and fatigue, are seen as a manifestation of this imbalance.

Herbal Remedies for Preventing Cold and Flu

Prevention is always better than cure, and traditional Chinese medicine offers several herbal remedies that can help prevent the onset of cold and flu.

Some of the most effective herbs for prevention include:

Ginseng (Ren Shen): Ginseng is a well-known adaptogen that helps to boost the immune system and increase resistance to disease. It is often used in combination with other herbs to prevent cold and flu.

Astragalus (Huang Qi): Astragalus is another adaptogen that is commonly used in traditional Chinese medicine to prevent cold and flu. It is believed to help stimulate the immune system and increase the body's natural defenses.

Echinacea (Mu Dan Pi): Echinacea is a popular herb that is often used to prevent cold and flu. It is believed to help stimulate the immune system and reduce the severity of symptoms.

Licorice Root (Glycyrrhizae): Licorice root is a natural expectorant that can help to relieve congestion and coughing. It is often used in combination with other herbs to prevent cold and flu.

Herbal Remedies for Treating Cold and Flu

While prevention is always the best approach, traditional Chinese medicine also offers several herbal remedies that can help treat cold and flu. Some of the most effective herbs for treatment include:

Ephedra (Ma Huang): Ephedra is a natural decongestant that can help to relieve congestion and coughing. It is often used in combination with other herbs to treat cold and flu.

Ginkgo Biloba (Bai Guo): Ginkgo biloba is a natural antiviral that can help to reduce the severity of cold and flu symptoms. It is believed to help stimulate the immune system and increase the body's natural defenses.

Schisandra (Wu Wei Zi): Schisandra is a natural antiviral that can help to reduce the severity of cold and flu symptoms. It is believed to help stimulate the immune system and increase the body's natural defenses.

Yarrow (Ding Xiang): Yarrow is a natural antiseptic that can help to reduce the severity of cold and flu symptoms. It is believed to help stimulate the immune system and increase the body's natural defenses.

Herbal Remedies for Digestive Problems such as Constipation and Diarrhea

In traditional Chinese medicine, digestive issues are often viewed as a manifestation of an imbalance in the body's energy, or "qi." This imbalance can be caused by a variety of factors, including poor diet, stress, and environmental toxins. Chinese herbal medicine offers a range of natural remedies that can help to restore balance to the digestive system and alleviate symptoms of constipation and diarrhea.

Constipation

Constipation is a common digestive issue that affects millions of people worldwide. It is characterized by infrequent bowel movements, hard stools, and straining during defecation. In traditional Chinese medicine, constipation is often viewed as a sign of stagnation in the digestive system, which can be caused by a variety of factors, including:

Poor diet: A diet that is high in processed foods, sugar, and dairy products can lead to constipation.

Stress: Stress can cause the body to produce more cortisol, which can slow down digestion and lead to constipation.

Environmental toxins: Exposure to environmental toxins, such as pesticides and heavy metals, can disrupt the digestive system and lead to constipation.

Chinese herbal medicine offers a range of natural remedies that can help to alleviate symptoms of constipation. Some of the most effective herbs for constipation include:

Rhubarb (Rhei radix): Rhubarb is a natural laxative that can help to stimulate bowel movements and relieve constipation

Glycyrrhizic acid (Glycyrrhizae radix): Glycyrrhizic acid is a natural anti-inflammatory that can help to soothe the digestive system and relieve symptoms of constipation.

Licorice root (Glycyrrhizae radix): Licorice root is a natural demulcent that can help to soothe the digestive system and relieve symptoms of constipation.

Dandelion root (Taraxaci radix): Dandelion root is a natural diuretic that can help to stimulate bowel movements and relieve constipation.

Diarrhea

Diarrhea is another common digestive issue that can be caused by a variety of factors, including:

Food poisoning: Eating contaminated food can lead to diarrhea.

Viral infections: Viral infections, such as the flu, can cause diarrhea.

Bacterial infections: Bacterial infections, such as giardiasis, can cause diarrhea.

Stress: Stress can cause the body to produce more cortisol, which can slow down digestion and lead to diarrhea.

Chinese herbal medicine offers a range of natural remedies that can help to alleviate symptoms of diarrhea.

Some of the most effective herbs for diarrhea include:

Ginger (Zingiberis rhizoma): Ginger is a natural anti-inflammatory that can help to soothe the digestive system and relieve symptoms of diarrhea.

Peppermint (Menthae piperitae): Peppermint is a natural antispasmodic that can help to relieve cramps and spasms in the digestive system and alleviate symptoms of diarrhea.

Licorice root (Glycyrrhizae radix): Licorice root is a natural demulcent that can help to soothe the digestive system and relieve symptoms of diarrhea.

Coptis (Coptidis rhizoma): Coptis is a natural antibacterial that can help to treat bacterial infections and alleviate symptoms of diarrhea.

Herbal Formulas

In addition to using individual herbs, Chinese herbal medicine also offers a range of herbal formulas that can be used to treat digestive issues such as constipation and diarrhea. Some of the most effective herbal formulas for digestive issues include:

Ba Zheng San: Ba Zheng San is a herbal formula that is used to treat constipation and other digestive issues. It is made from a combination of herbs, including *rhubarb, glycyrrhizic acid, and* *licorice root.*

Xiao Chai Hu Tang: Xiao Chai Hu Tang is a herbal formula that is used to treat diarrhea and other digestive issues. It is made from a combination of herbs, including *ginger, peppermint, and licorice root.*

Da Cheng Qi Tang: Da Cheng Qi Tang is a herbal formula that is used to treat constipation and other digestive issues. It is made from a combination of herbs, including *rhubarb, glycyrrhizic acid, and licorice root.*

Skin Conditions: Herbal Remedies for Acne and Eczema

In traditional Chinese medicine, the skin is believed to be a reflection of the body's internal balance and harmony. Skin conditions such as acne and eczema are often seen as a manifestation of an imbalance in the body's Qi, or vital energy. Chinese herbal medicine offers a range of remedies that can help to restore balance and alleviate symptoms of these conditions.

Acne

Acne is a common skin condition characterized by the formation of comedones (blackheads and whiteheads), papules, pustules, nodules, and cysts. In traditional Chinese medicine, acne is often attributed to an imbalance of the Liver and Stomach meridians, which can lead to the formation of heat and toxins in the body.

Herbal Remedies for Acne

Bai Zhi, also known as Angelica dahurica, Bai Zhi is a herb that is commonly used to treat acne. It is believed to have anti-inflammatory and antibacterial properties, which can help to reduce inflammation and prevent the growth of bacteria that can cause acne.

Huang Qin, also known as Cynanchum paniculatum, Huang Qin is a herb that is used to treat a range of skin conditions, including acne. It is believed to have anti-inflammatory and antioxidant properties, which can help to reduce inflammation and protect the skin from damage.

Xiang Fu, also known as Cyperus rotundus, Xiang Fu is a herb that is used to treat a range of skin conditions, including acne. It is believed to have anti-inflammatory and antibacterial properties, which can help to reduce inflammation and prevent the growth of bacteria that can cause acne.

Dang Gui, also known as Angelica sinensis, Dang Gui is a herb that is commonly used to treat a range of skin conditions, including acne. It is believed to have anti-inflammatory and antioxidant properties, which can help to reduce inflammation and protect the skin from damage.

Eczema

Eczema is a chronic skin condition characterized by dry, itchy, and inflamed skin. In traditional Chinese medicine, eczema is often attributed to an imbalance of the Lung and Spleen meridians, which can lead to the formation of dampness and heat in the body.

Herbal Remedies for Eczema

Huang Qi, also known as Astragalus membranaceus, Huang Qi is a herb that is commonly used to treat eczema. It is believed to have antiinflammatory and antioxidant properties, which can help to reduce inflammation and protect the skin from damage.

Bai Bu, also known as Dictamnus dasycarpus, Bai Bu is a herb that is used to treat a range of skin conditions, including eczema. It is believed to have anti-inflammatory and antibacterial properties, which can help to reduce inflammation and prevent the growth of bacteria that can cause eczema.

Ji Xue Teng, also known as Millettia nitida, Ji Xue Teng is a herb that is used to treat a range of skin conditions, including eczema. It is believed to have anti-inflammatory and antioxidant properties, which can help to reduce inflammation and protect the skin from damage.

Mu Dan Pi, also known as Moutan cortex, Mu Dan Pi is a herb that is commonly used to treat eczema. It is believed to have anti-inflammatory and antibacterial properties, which can help to reduce inflammation and prevent the growth of bacteria that can cause eczema.

Preparation and Administration

Herbal remedies for acne and eczema can be prepared in a variety of ways, including:

Decoction: Boiling the herbs in water to create a liquid extract.

Infusion: Steeping the herbs in hot water to create a liquid extract.

Powder: Grinding the herbs into a fine powder and mixing with water or other liquids.

Capsules: Encapsulating the herbs in a gelatin or vegetable-based capsule.

TCM Herbs in Modern Medicine

Traditional Chinese Medicine (TCM) has been practiced for thousands of years, and its herbal remedies have been an integral part of this ancient system of medicine. TCM herbs have been used to treat a wide range of health conditions, from common colds and flu to chronic diseases such as diabetes and cancer. In recent years, there has been a growing interest in the potential benefits of TCM herbs in modern medicine, and many studies have been conducted to investigate their efficacy and safety in treating health conditions including:

Cardiovascular disease: TCM herbs such as ginseng, astragalus, and licorice root have been shown to have potential benefits in reducing the risk of cardiovascular disease, including lowering blood pressure and cholesterol levels.

Cancer: TCM herbs such as turmeric, ginger, and green tea have been shown to have anti-cancer properties, and may be useful in preventing and treating cancer.

Diabetes: TCM herbs such as ginseng, astragalus, and licorice root have been shown to have potential benefits in managing blood sugar levels and improving insulin sensitivity.

Neurological disorders: TCM herbs such as ginkgo biloba, St. John's Wort, and valerian root have been shown to have potential benefits in treating neurological disorders such as Alzheimer's disease, Parkinson's disease, and depression.

Infectious diseases: TCM herbs such as echinacea, ginseng, and licorice root have been shown to have potential benefits in preventing and treating infectious diseases such as the common cold and flu.

7

Traditional Indian Medicine

Secrets of Ancient Indian Vedic Period: Herbal Remedies in Ancient India

The Vedic period, which spanned from approximately 1500 BCE to 500 BCE, was a time of great cultural and intellectual growth in ancient India. During this period, the Vedic civilization, which was centered in the Indo-Gangetic Plain, made significant contributions to the field of medicine, particularly in the use of herbal remedies. The Vedic people believed in the concept of "Ayurveda," which is a holistic approach to health that emphasizes the balance of the body's three doshas (vata, pitta, and kapha) and the use of natural remedies to prevent and treat diseases.

Herbs Used in Ancient India

The Vedic people used a wide variety of herbs to treat various ailments. Some of the most commonly used herbs included:

Turmeric (Curcuma longa): Turmeric was used to treat a range of conditions, including skin disorders, wounds, and digestive problems. It was also used as a natural dye and as a component of sacred rituals.

Ginger (Zingiber officinale): Ginger was used to treat digestive problems, nausea, and respiratory issues. It was also used as a natural remedy for colds and flu.

Neem (Azadirachta indica): Neem was used to treat a range of conditions, including skin disorders, fever, and digestive problems. It was also used as a natural insecticide and as a component of sacred rituals.

Ashwagandha (Withania somnifera): Ashwagandha was used to treat stress, anxiety, and insomnia. It was also used to improve cognitive function and to boost the immune system.

Basil (Ocimum sanctum): Basil was used to treat respiratory issues, such as bronchitis and asthma. It was also used to improve digestion and to reduce stress.

Guduchi (Tino spora cordifolia): Guduchi was used to treat fever, cough, and respiratory issues. It was also used to improve digestion and to boost the immune system.

Haridra (Curcuma longa): Haridra was used to treat skin disorders, wounds, and digestive problems. It was also used as a natural remedy for colds and flu.

Traditional Ayurvedic Medicine

The Vedic people believed that the key to good health was to maintain a balance between the body's three doshas. They used a variety of techniques, including herbal remedies, diet, and lifestyle changes, to achieve this balance. Ayurvedic medicine was based on the concept of "tridosha," which is the idea that the body is composed of three fundamental energies: vata, pitta, and kapha. Each of these energies was associated with specific characteristics, such as temperature, texture, and movement.

Vata Dosha: Vata is associated with the qualities of air and space. It is responsible for movement, communication, and creativity. Vata is also associated with the nervous system and the skin.

Pitta Dosha: Pitta is associated with the qualities of fire and water. It is responsible for digestion, metabolism, and energy. Pitta is also associated with the liver, spleen, and small intestine.

Kapha Dosha: Kapha is associated with the qualities of earth and water. It is responsible for structure, lubrication, and nourishment. Kapha is also associated with the lungs, throat, and sinuses.

Herbal Remedies in Ayurvedic Medicine

Ayurvedic medicine uses a variety of herbal remedies to treat a range of conditions. These remedies are based on the concept of "samanya" and "vishesha," which is the idea that each herb has a specific set of properties that can be used to treat specific conditions. Ayurvedic practitioners use a variety of techniques, including herbal remedies, diet, and lifestyle changes, to treat patients.

Samanya: Samanya refers to the general properties of a herb, such as its taste, texture, and temperature. Ayurvedic practitioners use samanya to determine the best way to use an herb to treat a specific condition.

Vishesha: Vishesha refers to the specific properties of a herb that are used to treat a specific condition. Ayurvedic practitioners use vishesha to determine the best way to use an herb to treat a specific condition.

Mughal Era

The Mughal era, which spanned from the early 16th century to the mid-18th century, was a period of significant cultural, economic, and artistic exchange between India and the rest of the world. The Mughal Empire, which was founded by Babur, a Central Asian ruler, was known for its rich cultural heritage, architectural achievements, and vibrant trade networks. During this period, India's herbal practices were influenced by foreign trade, leading to the introduction of new herbs, medicines, and treatment methods.

The Silk Road and the Spice Route

The Mughal Empire's strategic location at the crossroads of the Silk Road and the Spice Route made it an important hub for international trade. The Silk Road, which connected India to Central Asia, China, and the Mediterranean, was a major conduit for the exchange of goods, ideas, and cultures. The Spice Route, which connected India to Southeast Asia, the Middle East, and Europe, was a vital artery for the transportation of spices, textiles, and other valuable commodities.

As a result of this extensive trade network, India was exposed to a wide range of foreign herbs, spices, and medicines. Merchants and traders brought back exotic goods from their travels, which were then incorporated into Indian herbal practices. This influx of new herbs and medicines not only enriched India's pharmacopeia but also led to the development of new treatment methods and remedies.

Introduction of New Herbs

The Mughal era saw the introduction of several new herbs into Indian herbal practices. Some of the most significant imports included:

Turmeric (Curcuma longa): Turmeric, a spice commonly used in Indian cooking, was introduced to India from Southeast Asia during the Mughal era. It was used in traditional medicine to treat a range of ailments, including skin conditions, digestive problems, and wounds.

Ginger (Zingiber officinale): Ginger, another popular spice, was introduced to India from Southeast Asia during the Mughal era. It was used in traditional medicine to treat digestive problems, nausea, and respiratory issues.

Cardamom (Elettaria cardamomum): Cardamom, a spice commonly used in Indian cooking, was introduced to India from Southeast Asia during the Mughal era. It was used in traditional medicine to treat digestive problems, respiratory issues, and as a natural breath freshener.

Saffron (Crocus sativus): Saffron, a spice commonly used in Indian cooking, was introduced to India from the Middle East during the Mughal era. It was used in traditional medicine to treat a range of ailments, including digestive problems, respiratory issues, and as a natural dye.

Impact on Indian Herbal Practices

The introduction of new herbs during the Mughal era had a significant impact on Indian herbal practices. It led to the development of new treatment methods and remedies, as well as the creation of new herbal formulations. Some of the key ways in which foreign trade influenced Indian herbal practices include:

Synthesis of new remedies: The introduction of new herbs led to the synthesis of new remedies and treatment methods. For example, the combination of turmeric and ginger was used to treat digestive problems, while the combination of cardamom and saffron was used to treat respiratory issues.

Expansion of pharmacopeia: The introduction of new herbs expanded India's pharmacopeia, providing a wider range of options for treating various ailments. This expansion also led to the development of new herbal formulations and remedies.

Influence on Ayurvedic medicine: The introduction of new herbs during the Mughal era had a significant impact on Ayurvedic medicine, which is a traditional system of medicine that originated in India.

Ayurvedic practitioners incorporated new herbs into their treatments, leading to the development of new remedies and treatment methods.

British Colonization: Impact of Western Medicine

The British colonization of India, which lasted from the early 18th century to the mid-20th century, had a profound impact on the traditional herbology of the region. Prior to the arrival of the British, Indian traditional medicine, also known as Ayurveda, was a well-established and respected system of healing that had been practiced for thousands of years. Ayurveda relied heavily on the use of herbs, plants, and other natural substances to treat a wide range of ailments.

However, with the advent of British colonial rule, Western medicine began to gain prominence in India. The British introduced their own system of medicine, which was based on the principles of modern science and the use of pharmaceuticals. This led to a significant shift away from traditional Ayurvedic practices and towards the adoption of Western medicine.

One of the primary ways in which Western medicine impacted traditional herbology in India was through the introduction of new medical practices and treatments. The British established hospitals and medical schools in India, which trained Indian doctors in Western medical practices. This led to a decline in the use of traditional Ayurvedic remedies and an increase in the use of Western pharmaceuticals.

Another way in which Western medicine impacted traditional herbology was through the introduction of new herbs and plants. The British brought with them a wide range of plants and herbs from their own country, which were not native to India. These new plants and herbs were incorporated into Indian medicine, often replacing traditional Ayurvedic remedies.

Despite the impact of Western medicine on traditional herbology, many Indian doctors and healers continued to practice Ayurveda and use traditional remedies. In fact, Ayurveda has continued to thrive in India to this day, with many modern Indian doctors and healers incorporating traditional practices into their work. Some of the most commonly used herbs in Indian traditional medicine include:

Turmeric (Curcuma longa): Turmeric has been used for centuries in Indian medicine to treat a wide range of ailments, including digestive problems, skin conditions, and joint pain.

Ginger (Zingiber officinale): Ginger has been used in Indian medicine for centuries to treat digestive problems, nausea, and other ailments.

Neem (Azadirachta indica): Neem has been used in Indian medicine for centuries to treat a wide range of ailments, including skin conditions, digestive problems, and fever.

Ashwagandha (Withania somnifera): Ashwagandha has been used in Indian medicine for centuries to treat a wide range of ailments, including stress, anxiety, and insomnia.

Tulsi (Ocimum sanctum): Tulsi has been used in Indian medicine for centuries to treat a wide range of ailments, including colds, fever, and digestive problems.

These herbs, along with many others, continue to be used in Indian traditional medicine today. In fact, many modern Indian doctors and healers are incorporating traditional Ayurvedic remedies into their work, often in combination with Western medical practices.

Ayurvedic Herbs: Herbs used in traditional Indian medicine

Ayurveda, the ancient Indian system of medicine, has been using herbs for thousands of years to promote health, prevent disease, and treat various ailments. The use of herbs in Ayurveda is based on the concept of "tridosha" or the three fundamental energies of the body - Vata, Pitta, and Kapha. Each herb is believed to have a specific action on one or more of these doshas, and is used to restore balance to the body and maintain overall health.

1. Turmeric (Curcuma longa) Turmeric is one of the most widely used herbs in Ayurveda, and is considered a "rasayana" or a rejuvenating herb. It is believed to have anti-inflammatory, antioxidant, and antibacterial properties, and is used to treat a variety of conditions, including arthritis, digestive disorders, and skin problems.

Properties: Turmeric is a warm herb that is believed to increase Pitta and Kapha doshas, while reducing Vata dosha.

Uses:

Digestive disorders: Turmeric is used to treat digestive disorders such as bloating, gas, and indigestion.

Arthritis: Turmeric is used to treat arthritis, including osteoarthritis and rheumatoid arthritis.

Skin problems: Turmeric is used to treat skin problems such as acne, eczema, and psoriasis.

Wound healing: Turmeric is used to promote wound healing and reduce the risk of infection.

2. Ginger (Zingiber officinale)Ginger is another commonly used herb in Ayurveda, and is believed to have anti-inflammatory, antioxidant, and antibacterial properties. It is used to treat a variety of conditions, including digestive disorders, nausea, and respiratory problems.

<u>Properties</u>: Ginger is a warm herb that is believed to increase Pitta and Kapha doshas, while reducing Vata dosha.

<u>Uses</u>:

Digestive disorders: Ginger is used to treat digestive disorders such as bloating, gas, and indigestion.

Nausea: Ginger is used to treat nausea and vomiting, including morning sickness during pregnancy.

Respiratory problems: Ginger is used to treat respiratory problems such as bronchitis, asthma, and coughs.

Pain relief: Ginger is used to treat pain, including menstrual cramps and arthritis.

3. Ashwagandha (Withania somnifera)

Ashwagandha is an adaptogenic herb that is believed to help the body adapt to stress and promote overall health. It is used to treat a variety of conditions, including anxiety, insomnia, and fatigue.

<u>Properties</u>: Ashwagandha is a warm herb that is believed to increase Vata and Kapha doshas, while reducing Pitta dosha.

<u>Uses</u>:

Stress relief: Ashwagandha is used to treat stress, anxiety, and insomnia.

Fatigue: Ashwagandha is used to treat fatigue and weakness.

Menstrual problems: Ashwagandha is used to treat menstrual problems such as cramps, bloating, and mood swings.

Immune system: Ashwagandha is used to boost the immune system and prevent illness.

4. Triphala (Terminalia chebula, Terminalia belerica, and Emblica officinalis)

Triphala is a combination of three herbs - Amalaki, Haritaki, and Bibhitaki - that is believed to promote overall health and well-being. It is used to treat a variety of conditions, including digestive disorders, respiratory problems, and skin problems.

Properties: Triphala is a cooling herb that is believed to balance all three doshas - Vata, Pitta, and Kapha.

Uses:

Digestive disorders: Triphala is used to treat digestive disorders such as constipation, diarrhea, and bloating.

Respiratory problems: Triphala is used to treat respiratory problems such as bronchitis, asthma, and coughs.

Skin problems: Triphala is used to treat skin problems such as acne, eczema, and psoriasis.

Eye problems: Triphala is used to treat eye problems such as conjunctivitis and cataracts.

5. Neem (Azadirachta indica)

Neem is a tree that is believed to have antibacterial, antiviral, and antifungal properties. It is used to treat a variety of conditions, including skin problems,

respiratory problems, and digestive disorders.

Properties: Neem is a cooling herb that is believed to reduce all three doshas - Vata, Pitta, and Kapha.

Uses: Skin problems: Neem is used to treat skin problems such as acne, eczema, and psoriasis.

Respiratory problems: Neem is used to treat respiratory problems such as bronchitis, asthma, and coughs.

Digestive disorders: Neem is used to treat digestive disorders such as bloating, gas, and indigestion.

Hair and scalp problems: Neem is used to treat hair and scalp problems such as dandruff and hair loss.

6. Giloy (Tinospora cordifolia)

Giloy is a herb that is believed to have anti-inflammatory,

antioxidant, and antibacterial properties. It is used to treat a variety of conditions, including fever, cough, and digestive disorders.

<u>Properties</u>: Giloy is a warm herb that is believed to increase Pitta and Kapha doshas, while reducing Vata dosha.

<u>Uses</u>:

Fever: Giloy is used to treat fever and reduce body temperature.

Cough: Giloy is used to treat cough and reduce inflammation in the throat.

Digestive disorders: Giloy is used to treat digestive disorders such as bloating, gas, and indigestion.

Skin problems: Giloy is used to treat skin problems such as acne, eczema, and psoriasis.

7. *Guggulu* (Commiphora mukul)

Guggulu is a resin that is believed to have anti-inflammatory, antioxidant, and antibacterial properties. It is used to treat a variety of conditions, including arthritis, digestive disorders, and skin problems.

<u>Properties</u>: Guggulu is a warm herb that is believed to increase Pitta and Kapha doshas, while reducing Vata dosha.

<u>Uses</u>:

Arthritis: Guggulu is used to treat arthritis, including osteoarthritis and rheumatoid arthritis.

Digestive disorders: Guggulu is used to treat digestive disorders such as bloating, gas, and indigestion.

Skin problems: Guggulu is used to treat skin problems such as acne, eczema, and psoriasis.

Wound healing: Guggulu is used to promote wound healing and reduce the risk of infection.

8. *Haritaki* (Terminalia chebula)

Haritaki is a herb that is believed to have anti-inflammatory, antioxidant, and antibacterial properties. It is used to treat a variety of conditions, including digestive disorders, respiratory problems, and skin problems.

Properties: Haritaki is a cooling herb that is believed to balance all three doshas - Vata, Pitta, and Kapha.

Uses:

Digestive disorders: Haritaki is used to treat digestive disorders such as constipation, diarrhea, and bloating.

Respiratory problems: Haritaki is used to treat respiratory problems such as bronchitis, asthma, and coughs.

Skin problems: Haritaki is used to treat skin problems such as acne, eczema, and psoriasis.

Eye problems: Haritaki is used to treat eye problems such as conjunctivitis and cataracts.

9. *Bibhitaki* (Terminalia belerica)

Bibhitaki is a herb that is believed to have anti-inflammatory, antioxidant, and antibacterial properties. It is used to treat a variety of conditions, including digestive disorders, respiratory problems, and skin problems.

Properties: Bibhitaki is a cooling herb that is believed to balance all three doshas - Vata, Pitta, and Kapha.

Uses:

Digestive disorders: Bibhitaki is used to treat digestive disorders such as constipation, diarrhea, and bloating.

Respiratory problems: Bibhitaki is used to treat respiratory problems such as bronchitis, asthma, and coughs.

Skin problems: Bibhitaki is used to treat skin problems such as acne, eczema, and psoriasis.

Eye problems: Bibhitaki is used to treat eye problems such as conjunctivitis and cataracts.

10. Amalaki (Emblica officinalis)

Amalaki is a herb that is believed to have anti-inflammatory, antioxidant, and antibacterial properties. It is used to treat a variety of conditions, including digestive disorders, respiratory problems, and skin problems.

<u>Properties</u>: Amalaki is a cooling herb that is believed to balance all three doshas - Vata, Pitta, and Kapha.

<u>Uses</u>:

Digestive disorders: Amalaki is used to treat digestive disorders such as constipation, diarrhea, and bloating.

Respiratory problems: Amalaki is used to treat respiratory problems such as bronchitis, asthma, and coughs.

Skin problems: Amalaki is used to treat skin problems such as acne, eczema, and psoriasis.

Eye problems: Amalaki is used to treat eye problems such as conjunctivitis and cataracts.

Herbs used in Unani Medicine

Unani medicine is another traditional system of medicine that originated in India. It is based on the concept of humoral theory, which posits that the body contains four humors: blood, phlegm, yellow bile, and black bile. Unani practitioners use herbs to balance and restore the humors, which is believed to promote overall health and well-being. Some of the most commonly used herbs in Unani medicine include:

Guggul (Commiphora mukul): Guggul is used to treat a range of conditions, including arthritis, digestive issues, and skin problems. Its anti-inflammatory and antioxidant properties make it a popular ingredient in Unani remedies.

Saffron (Crocus sativus): Saffron is used to treat a range of conditions, including depression, anxiety, and insomnia.

Fenugreek (Trigonella foenum-graecum): Fenugreek is used to treat digestive issues, respiratory problems, and skin problems.

Herbs used in Siddha Medicine

Siddha medicine is a traditional system of medicine that originated in southern India. It is based on the concept of three humors: vata, pitta, and kapha. Siddha practitioners use herbs to balance and restore the humors, which is believed to promote overall health and well-being. Some of the most commonly used herbs in Siddha medicine include:

Aloe vera (Aloe barbadensis): Aloe vera is used to treat a range of conditions, including skin problems, digestive issues, and respiratory problems. Its anti-inflammatory and antioxidant properties make it a popular ingredient in Siddha remedies.

Guduchi (Tinospora cordifolia): Guduchi is used to treat a range of conditions, including fever, cough, and skin problems.

Haridra (Curcuma longa): Haridra is used to treat a range of conditions, including arthritis, digestive issues, and skin problems.

Herbs for Digestive Issues: Natural Solutions for Gut Health

Digestive issues are a common problem that affects millions of people worldwide. From bloating and cramps to diarrhea and constipation, the symptoms can be uncomfortable and debilitating. While conventional medicine often relies on pharmaceuticals to treat these issues, many people are turning to natural remedies, including herbs, to promote gut health and alleviate digestive problems.

Ayurvedic Herbs for Digestive Issues

Ayurvedic medicine, which originated in India over 3,000 years ago, places a strong emphasis on the importance of digestive health. According to Ayurvedic philosophy, the digestive system is responsible for breaking down food and absorbing nutrients, and any imbalance in the digestive system can lead to a range of health problems. Ayurvedic practitioners have developed a range of herbal remedies to promote digestive health and alleviate digestive issues.

*1. **Triphala*** Triphala is a combination of three herbs - Amalaki (Emblica officinalis),

Haritaki (Terminalia chebula), and Bibhitaki (Terminalia bellirica) - that is commonly used in Ayurvedic medicine to promote digestive health. Triphala is believed to have anti-inflammatory and antioxidant properties, which can help to soothe the digestive tract and reduce inflammation. Studies have shown that Triphala can help to alleviate symptoms of irritable bowel syndrome (IBS), including bloating, abdominal pain, and changes in bowel habits.

2. *Ginger* (Zingiber officinale) is another herb that has been used for centuries in Ayurvedic medicine to treat digestive issues. Ginger has anti-inflammatory properties that can help to reduce inflammation in the digestive tract, which can alleviate symptoms of IBS and other digestive disorders. Ginger has also been shown to have antioxidant properties, which can help to protect the digestive system from damage caused by free radicals.

3. *Turmeric* (Curcuma longa) is a spice that has been used for centuries in Indian cuisine and Ayurvedic medicine. Turmeric contains a compound called curcumin, which has potent anti-inflammatory and antioxidant properties. Curcumin has been shown to reduce inflammation in the digestive tract, which can alleviate symptoms of IBS and other digestive disorders. Turmeric has also been shown to have antimicrobial properties, which can help to prevent the growth of harmful bacteria in the digestive system.

4. *Neem* (Azadirachta indica) is a tree that has been used for centuries in Ayurvedic medicine to treat a range of health problems, including digestive issues. Neem has anti-inflammatory and antioxidant properties that can help to soothe the digestive tract and reduce inflammation. Neem has also been shown to have antimicrobial properties, which can help to prevent the growth of harmful bacteria in the digestive system.

5. *Cumin* (Cuminum cyminum) is a spice that is commonly used in Indian cuisine and Ayurvedic medicine. Cumin has anti-inflammatory properties that can help to reduce inflammation in the digestive tract, which can alleviate symptoms of IBS and other digestive disorders. Cumin has also been shown to have antioxidant properties, which can help to protect the digestive system from damage caused by free radicals.

*6. **Coriander*** (Coriandrum sativum) is a spice that is commonly used in Indian cuisine and Ayurvedic medicine. Coriander has anti-inflammatory properties that can help to reduce inflammation in the digestive tract, which can alleviate symptoms of IBS and other digestive disorders. Coriander has also been shown to have antioxidant properties, which can help to protect the digestive system from damage caused by free radicals.

Herbs for Skin Problems: Herbal Remedies for Skin Conditions

In the ancient tradition of Ayurvedic medicine, herbs have been used for centuries to treat a wide range of skin conditions. The Indian subcontinent, with its rich cultural heritage and diverse flora, has been a treasure trove of herbal remedies for skin problems. In this chapter, we will explore the various herbs used in India to treat skin conditions, their properties, and their applications.

Ayurvedic Perspective on Skin

In Ayurveda, the skin is considered to be the largest organ of the body, and its health is closely linked to overall well-being. The skin is seen as a reflection of the body's internal balance, and imbalances in the body's doshas (Vata, Pitta, and Kapha) can manifest as skin problems. Ayurvedic practitioners believe that the skin is a dynamic system that is constantly interacting with the environment, and that herbal remedies can be used to restore balance and promote healthy skin.

Turmeric (Curcuma longa): Turmeric is one of the most

widely used herbs in Ayurvedic medicine for skin problems. Its anti-inflammatory and antioxidant properties make it an effective treatment for acne, eczema, and other skin conditions. Turmeric is also used to treat skin infections, wounds, and burns.

Properties: Anti-inflammatory, antioxidant, antibacterial

Applications: Acne, eczema, skin infections, wounds, burns.

Neem (Azadirachta indica): Neem is a versatile herb that has been used for centuries in Ayurvedic medicine to treat a range of skin conditions, including acne, eczema, and skin infections. Its antibacterial and antifungal properties make it an effective treatment for skin problems caused by fungal and bacterial infections.

Properties: Antibacterial, antifungal, anti-inflammatory

Applications: Acne, eczema, skin infections, fungal infections

Aloe Vera (Aloe barbadensis): Aloe vera is a popular herb that has been used for centuries to treat skin problems, including burns, wounds, and skin conditions such as eczema and acne. Its anti-inflammatory and antioxidant properties make it an effective treatment for skin irritations and injuries.

Properties: Anti-inflammatory, antioxidant, soothing

Applications: Burns, wounds, eczema, acne, skin irritations

Ginger (Zingiber officinale): Ginger is a commonly used herb in Ayurvedic medicine that has anti-inflammatory and antioxidant properties, making it an effective treatment for skin conditions such as acne, eczema, and skin infections.

Properties: Anti-inflammatory, antioxidant, antibacterial

Applications: Acne, eczema, skin infections, digestive issues

Fenugreek (Trigonella foenum-graecum): Fenugreek is a herb that has been used for centuries in Ayurvedic medicine to treat skin conditions such as eczema, acne, and skin infections.

Its antiinflammatory and antioxidant properties make it an effective treatment for skin problems caused by inflammation and oxidative stress.

<u>Properties</u>: Anti-inflammatory, antioxidant, antibacterial

<u>Applications</u>: Eczema, acne, skin infections, digestive issues

Bhringaraj (Eclipta alba): Bhringaraj is a herb that has been used for centuries in Ayurvedic medicine to treat skin conditions such as leucoderma, a condition characterized by white patches on the skin. Its antioxidant and anti-inflammatory properties make it an effective treatment for skin problems caused by oxidative stress and inflammation.

<u>Properties</u>: Antioxidant, anti-inflammatory, antibacterial

<u>Applications</u>: Leucoderma, skin infections, wounds, burns

Haridra (Curcuma longa): Haridra is a herb that has been used for centuries in Ayurvedic medicine to treat skin conditions such as acne, eczema, and skin infections. Its anti-inflammatory and antioxidant properties make it an effective treatment for skin problems caused by inflammation and oxidative stress.

<u>Properties</u>: Anti-inflammatory, antioxidant, antibacterial

<u>Applications</u>: Acne, eczema, skin infections, digestive issues

Herbs for Respiratory Issues: Natural treatments for colds and coughs

In the ancient traditions of Ayurvedic medicine, herbs have been used for centuries to treat a wide range of respiratory issues, from common colds and coughs to chronic bronchitis and asthma. The Indian subcontinent, in particular, has a rich heritage of herbal remedies that have been passed down through generations, offering a natural and effective way to alleviate respiratory distress.

The Ayurvedic Perspective

The respiratory system is considered to be closely linked to the doshas, or the three fundamental energies that govern the body. The doshas are Vata, Pitta, and Kapha, and each is associated with specific characteristics and functions. When the doshas become imbalanced, it can lead to a range of respiratory issues, from congestion and coughing to wheezing and shortness of breath.

Herbs for Colds and Coughs

When it comes to treating colds and coughs, Ayurvedic medicine offers a range of herbs that can help to alleviate symptoms and promote recovery. Some of the most commonly used herbs include:

Tulsi (Ocimum sanctum): Also known as holy basil, tulsi is a natural expectorant that helps to loosen and clear mucus from the lungs. It is often used in combination with other herbs to treat respiratory infections and allergies.

Ginger (Zingiber officinale): Ginger has natural anti-inflammatory properties that can help to reduce congestion and soothe a sore throat. It is often used in tea form, either on its own or in combination with other herbs.

Echinacea (Echinacea spp.): Echinacea is a flowering plant that is native to North America, but is also commonly used in Ayurvedic medicine. It is believed to have immune-boosting properties that can help to prevent and treat respiratory infections.

Turmeric (Curcuma longa): Turmeric contains a powerful anti inflammatory compound called curcumin, which can help to reduce inflammation and congestion in the lungs. It is often used in combination with other herbs to treat respiratory issues.

Herbs for Chronic Respiratory Issues

In addition to treating colds and coughs, Ayurvedic medicine also offers a range of herbs that can help to alleviate symptoms of chronic respiratory issues, such as bronchitis and asthma. Some of the most commonly used herbs include:

Adaptogenic herbs: Herbs such as ashwagandha (Withania somnifera) and brahmi (Bacopa monnieri) are believed to have adaptogenic properties that can help to reduce stress and anxiety, which can exacerbate respiratory issues.

Expectorant herbs: Herbs such as licorice root (Glycyrrhiza glabra) and thyme (Thymus vulgaris) are natural expectorants that can help to loosen and clear mucus from the lungs.

Antispasmodic herbs: Herbs such as ginger and turmeric are believed to have antispasmodic properties that can help to relax the airways and reduce wheezing and coughing.

Preparing Herbs for Respiratory Issues

In Ayurvedic medicine, herbs are often prepared in a variety of ways to enhance their effectiveness and bioavailability. Some common methods include:

Tea: Herbs can be steeped in hot water to make a soothing tea that can be consumed several times a day.

Decoction: Herbs can be simmered in water for a longer period of time to extract their active compounds and create a more concentrated remedy.

Poultice: Herbs can be applied topically as a poultice to help reduce inflammation and congestion in the lungs.

Capsules: Herbs can be encapsulated in a powdered form to make it easier to consume and ensure consistent dosing.

Types of Herbs Used in Ayurveda

Rasayana Herbs: These herbs are used to promote overall health and well-being, and are believed to have anti-aging properties. Examples of Rasayana herbs include Ashwagandha, Amalaki, and Haridra.

Medhya Herbs: These herbs are used to improve mental clarity, memory, and cognitive function. Examples of Medhya herbs include Brahmi, Jatamansi, and Shankapushpi.

Vata-Pacifying Herbs: These herbs are used to balance Vata dosha and are believed to have a calming effect on the nervous system. Examples of Vata-pacifying herbs include Ashwagandha, Jatamansi, and Tagar.

Pitta-Pacifying Herbs: These herbs are used to balance Pitta dosha and are believed to have a cooling effect on the body. Examples of Pittapacifying herbs include Amla, Haridra, and Manjishtha.

Kapha-Pacifying Herbs: These herbs are used to balance Kapha dosha and are believed to have a warming effect on the body. Examples of Kapha-pacifying herbs include Triphala, Haridra, and Kutki.

Herbal Remedies in Unani Medicine: The Influence of Greek Medicine on Indian Herbology

Unani medicine, also known as Yunani medicine, is a system of traditional medicine that originated in ancient Greece and was later adopted and adapted in India. The term "Unani" is derived from the Greek word "Ionian," which refers to the Ionian region of Greece. Unani medicine is based on the principles of Greek medicine, particularly the teachings of Galen and Hippocrates, and has been practiced in India for centuries. One of the key components of Unani medicine is the use of herbal remedies. Herbal remedies have been used in India for thousands of years, and were an integral part of the traditional medicine practiced in the region. The use of herbs in Unani medicine is based on the concept of "Tibb-e-Nabawi," which is the study of the natural remedies used by the Prophet Muhammad. According to this concept, herbs are considered to be a gift from God, and are used to treat a wide range of health conditions.

The use of herbal remedies in Unani medicine is influenced by the Greek concept of "humorism," which is the idea that the body is composed of four fluid-like substances, or "humors," that must be kept in balance in order to maintain good health. The four humors are blood, phlegm, yellow bile, and black bile, and they are associated with different seasons, temperatures, and environments. The use of herbal remedies in Unani medicine is based on the idea that certain herbs can help to balance the humors and restore health to the body.

The Influence of Greek Medicine on Indian Herbology

The use of herbal remedies in Unani medicine is heavily influenced by the teachings of Greek medicine. The Greek physician Galen, who lived in the 2nd century AD, is considered to be one of the most important figures in the history of Unani medicine. Galen's teachings on the use of herbal remedies were widely adopted in India, and his writings on the subject are still studied by Unani practitioners today.

One of the key concepts that Greek medicine introduced to Indian herbology is the idea of "similia similibus curantur," which is the idea that like cures like. This concept is based on the idea that a substance that produces a particular effect on the body can also be used to cure a condition that is characterized by that effect. For example, if a substance causes a fever, it can also be used to treat a fever. This concept is still used in Unani medicine today, and is an important part of the way that herbal remedies are selected and used.

Another important concept that Greek medicine introduced to Indian herbology is the idea of "contraria contrariis curantur," which is the idea that opposites cure opposites. This concept is based on the idea that a substance that has an opposite effect to a particular condition can be used to cure that condition. For example, if a substance has a cooling effect, it can be used to treat a condition that is characterized by heat. This concept is also still used in Unani medicine today, and is an important part of the way that herbal remedies are selected and used.

8

African Tribes, Native Cultures

Herbalism has been an integral part of African culture for centuries, with various tribes and native cultures utilizing plants and herbs for medicinal, spiritual, and culinary purposes. The use of herbs in Africa dates back to ancient times, with evidence of herbal remedies found in the earliest recorded history of the continent.

Early History of Herbalism in Africa

The earliest recorded use of herbs in Africa dates back to around 3000 BCE, during the Neolithic period. Archaeological findings in the Nile Valley and other parts of Africa have revealed evidence of herbal remedies, including the use of plants for medicinal and spiritual purposes. The ancient Egyptians, for example, used herbs such as *chamomile, lavender, and mint* for their calming and soothing properties, while the ancient Nubians used herbs like *aloe vera and papyrus* for their medicinal and spiritual significance. Traditional Use of

Herbs in African Tribes Herbalism played a significant role in the daily lives of African tribes, with each tribe having its own unique tradition and approach to using herbs. In many African cultures, herbalism was passed down from generation to generation, with elders and spiritual leaders serving as the primary authorities on herbal remedies. In West Africa, for example, the Yoruba people of Nigeria used herbs like *senna, bitter leaf, and ginger* to treat a range of ailments, including fever, cough, and digestive issues. The Ashanti people of Ghana, on the other hand, used herbs like *neem, basil, and lemongrass* to treat skin conditions, wounds, and respiratory problems. In East Africa, the Maasai people of Kenya and Tanzania used herbs like *chamomile, lavender, and rosemary* to treat anxiety, insomnia, and digestive issues. The Maasai people also used herbs like a*loe vera and papyrus* to treat skin conditions and wounds.

Native Cultures in Africa, such as the San people of Southern Africa, also played a significant role in the use of herbs. The San people used herbs like *devil's claw, cape aloe, and bushwillow* to treat a range of ailments, including fever, cough, and digestive issues. The San people also used herbs like *chamomile and lavender* to treat anxiety and insomnia. Herbalism played a major role in African society, with herbs being used for a range of purposes beyond just medicine.

Herbalism also played a significant role in African economic and social systems, with many communities relying on herbal remedies as a primary source of healthcare. In many cases, herbal remedies were more accessible and affordable than modern medicine, making them a vital part of African healthcare systems.

Africa is home to a vast array of herbs, with over 10,000 plant species being used in traditional medicine alone. From the deserts of North Africa to the rainforests of Central and West Africa, herbs like chamomile, lavender and rosemary are used to treat a range of ailments, including fever, cough, and digestive issues.

In East Africa, herbs like *neem, basil, and lemongrass* are used to treat skin conditions, wounds, and respiratory problems. In Southern Africa, herbs like *devil's claw, cape aloe and bushwillow* are used to treat fever, cough and digestive issues.

There are several challenges facing the traditional use of herbs in Africa. One of the main challenges is the lack of formal recognition and regulation of traditional herbal medicine, which can make it difficult for communities to access and use herbal remedies. Another challenge is the impact of globalization and modernization on traditional herbal practices, with many communities abandoning their traditional practices in favor of modern medicine. This can lead to a loss of cultural heritage and traditional knowledge, as well as a decline in the use of herbal remedies.

Herbal Remedies for Common Ailments

Herbal remedies have been used for centuries to treat a wide range of common ailments and injuries. These remedies are often based on traditional knowledge passed down through generations, and are often more effective and safer than modern pharmaceuticals.

Respiratory Issues

Respiratory issues such as bronchitis, asthma, and the common cold are common in many parts of the world. In African tribes and Native cultures, several herbs are used to treat these conditions. One of the most effective herbs is *Echinacea*, which is used to boost the immune system and reduce inflammation in the lungs. Another herb commonly used is *Marshmallow root,* which soothes the throat and reduces coughing. In the Amazon rainforest, the indigenous people use the leaves of the *"Pau d'Arco"* tree to treat respiratory issues. The leaves are made into a tea that is rich in antioxidants and has anti-inflammatory properties. In Africa, the *"African Ginger"* plant is used to treat respiratory issues. The roots of the plant are made into a tea that is warm and spicy, and is used to relieve congestion and coughing.

Digestive Issues

Digestive issues such as diarrhea, constipation, and indigestion are common in many parts of the world. In African tribes and Native cultures, several herbs are used to treat these conditions. One of the most effective herbs is *Slippery Elm*, which soothes the digestive tract and reduces inflammation. Another herb commonly used is *Ginger*, which reduces nausea and relieves digestive discomfort. In the Andes mountains, the indigenous people use the leaves of the *"Quinoa"* plant to treat digestive issues. The leaves are made into a tea that is rich in fiber and has anti-inflammatory properties. In Africa, the *"Buchu"* plant is used to treat digestive issues. The leaves of the plant are made into a tea that is warm and spicy, and is used to relieve digestive discomfort and reduce inflammation.

Infections and Wounds

Infections and wounds are common in many parts of the world. In African tribes and Native cultures, several herbs are used to treat these conditions. One of the most effective herbs is *Tea Tree oil*, which has antibacterial and antifungal properties. Another herb commonly used is *Calendula*, which promotes healing and reduces inflammation. In the Amazon rainforest, the indigenous people use the sap of the *"Dragon's Blood" tree* to treat infections and wounds. The sap is rich in antioxidants and has antibacterial properties. In Africa, the *"Aloe Vera"* plant is used to treat infections and wounds. The gel of the plant is applied topically to promote healing and reduce inflammation.

Pain Relief

Is a common need in many parts of the world. In African tribes and Native cultures, several herbs are used to treat pain. One of the most effective herbs is *Willow bark*, which contains salicin, a natural pain reliever. Another herb commonly used is *Turmeric*, which reduces inflammation and relieves pain. In the Andes mountains, the indigenous people use the roots of the *"Coca" plant* to treat pain. The roots are made into a tea that is rich in alkaloids and has analgesic properties. In Africa, the *"Devil's Claw"* plant is used to treat pain. The roots of the plant are made into a tea that is warm and spicy, and is used to relieve pain and reduce inflammation.

Menstrual Relief

In African tribes and Native cultures, several herbs are used to treat menstrual cramps, bloating, and mood swings. One of the most effective herbs is *Chamomile*, which soothes the uterus and reduces inflammation. Another herb commonly used is *Red Clover*, which reduces bloating and relieves menstrual cramps. In the Amazon rainforest, the indigenous people use the leaves of the *"Piper Methysticum"* plant to treat menstrual relief. The leaves are made into a tea that is rich in alkaloids and has anti-inflammatory properties. In Africa, the *"Sida Cordifolia"* plant is used to treat menstrual relief. The leaves of the plant are made into a tea that is warm and spicy, and is used to relieve menstrual cramps and reduce bloating.

Herbs Healing Properties of African Herbs:

Various African Herbs have been used for centuries to treat various ailments and diseases. The continent is home to a diverse range of flora, with many plants possessing unique medicinal properties.

*1. **Sickle Bush*** (Dorstenia barteri), also known as "Nsoko" in some African cultures, is a plant native to West Africa. Its leaves, stems, and roots are used to treat various health conditions, including: *Fever:* The plant's leaves are used to reduce fever and alleviate symptoms of malaria. *Skin conditions:* The plant's roots are used to treat skin conditions such as eczema, acne, and dermatitis. *Digestive issues:* The plant's leaves are used to treat digestive issues such as diarrhea, constipation, and stomach pain.

*2. **African Ginger*** (Zingiber officinale), also known as "Ginger" or "Kunyit" in some African cultures, is a plant native to West Africa. Its rhizomes are used to treat various health conditions, including: *Digestive issues:* The plant's rhizomes are used to treat digestive issues such as nausea, vomiting, and stomach pain. *Inflammation:* The plant's rhizomes are used to reduce inflammation and alleviate symptoms of arthritis. *Respiratory issues:* The plant's rhizomes are used to treat respiratory issues such as bronchitis and asthma.

*3. **Baobab Tree*** (Adansonia digitata)is a plant native to Africa, with its bark, leaves, and seeds used to treat various health conditions, including: *Digestive issues:* The plant's bark is used to treat digestive issues such as diarrhea, constipation, and stomach pain. *Skin conditions:* The plant's leaves are used to treat skin conditions such as eczema, acne, and dermatitis. *Respiratory issues:* The plant's seeds are used to treat respiratory issues such as bronchitis and asthma.

4. African Basil (Ocimum kilimandscharicum), also known as "Sweet Basil" or "Kilimandscharicum" in some African cultures, is a plant native to East Africa. Its leaves are used to treat various health conditions, including: *Digestive issues:* The plant's leaves are used to treat digestive issues such as nausea, vomiting, and stomach pain.

Inflammation: The plant's leaves are used to reduce inflammation and alleviate symptoms of arthritis. *Respiratory issues:* The plant's leaves are used to treat respiratory issues such as bronchitis and asthma.

*5. **Devil's Claw*** (Harpagophytum procumbens), also known as "Grapple Plant" or "Harpagophytum" in some African cultures, is a plant native to Southern Africa. Its roots are used to treat various health conditions, including: *Pain relief:* The plant's roots are used to treat pain and alleviate symptoms of arthritis. *Inflammation:* The plant's roots are used to reduce inflammation and alleviate symptoms of gout. *Digestive issues:* The plant's roots are used to treat digestive issues such as diarrhea, constipation, and stomach pain.

6. African Marigold (Tagetes erecta), also known as "Kikoye" in some African cultures, is a plant native to West Africa. Its flowers are used to treat various health conditions, including: *Skin conditions:* The plant's flowers are used to treat skin

conditions such as eczema, acne, and dermatitis. *Digestive issues:* The plant's flowers are used to treat digestive issues such as diarrhea, constipation, and stomach pain. *Respiratory issues:* The plant's flowers are used to treat respiratory issues such as bronchitis and asthma.

7. Ginger (Zingiber officinale), also known as "Kunyit" in some African cultures, is a plant native to West Africa. Its rhizomes are used to treat various health conditions, including: *Digestive issues:* The plant's rhizomes are used to treat digestive issues such as nausea, vomiting, and stomach pain. *Inflammation:* The plant's rhizomes are used to reduce inflammation and alleviate symptoms of arthritis. *Respiratory issues:* The plant's rhizomes are used to treat respiratory issues such as bronchitis and asthma.

Herbalism in Traditional African Medicine

Traditional African medicine, also known as "traditional healing," is a holistic approach to healthcare that emphasizes the use of natural remedies, including herbs to treat a wide range of ailments. Herbalism is a key component of traditional African medicine, with many herbs being used to treat conditions such as fever, cough, and skin infections. The use of herbs in traditional African medicine is often tied to the concept of "hot" and "cold" energies, with certain herbs being used to balance and harmonize the body's energies. The Use of Herbs in African Rituals and Ceremonies Herbs play a significant role in many African rituals and ceremonies, including initiation ceremonies, weddings, and funerals. In these contexts, herbs are often used to purify, protect, and consecrate individuals, spaces, and objects. For example, in some African cultures, herbs are used to purify the body and spirit before initiation into a spiritual or cultural tradition. In other cultures, herbs are used to protect individuals from harm and evil spirits.

The Importance of Herbalism in African Culture

Herbalism is an important part of African culture, with many herbs being used in traditional medicine, rituals, and ceremonies. The use of herbs is often tied to the concept of community and shared knowledge, with herbal remedies being passed down from generation to generation. Herbalism is also an important part of African spirituality, with many herbs being used to connect with the divine, honor ancestors, and promote spiritual growth.

Herbal Traditions in West Africa

West Africa is home to a rich cultural heritage, with a long history of traditional medicine and herbalism. The region's diverse ethnic groups have developed unique systems of healing, often relying on the use of plants, roots, and other natural substances to treat a wide range of ailments.

The Cultural Significance of Herbalism in West Africa

Herbalism is deeply ingrained in West African culture, with many communities relying on traditional medicine as their primary source of healthcare. In many cases, herbal remedies are passed down from generation to generation, with knowledge and skills being transmitted orally from elder to younger generations. Herbalism is often seen as a way of connecting with one's ancestors and cultural heritage, and is closely tied to spiritual and religious practices. In West Africa, herbalism is often practiced by traditional healers, known as "herbalists" or "doctors." These individuals have spent years studying and learning about the properties and uses of various plants, and are highly • respected within their communities for their knowledge and skills. Herbalists may use a combination of plant-based remedies, spiritual practices, and other traditional techniques to diagnose and treat a wide range of health conditions.

Types of Plants Used in West African Herbalism

West Africa is home to a vast array of plant species, many of which have been used for centuries in traditional medicine. Some of the most commonly used plants include:

African Mango (Irvingia gabonensis): Also known as "ogbono," this plant is used to treat a range of health conditions, including fever, rheumatism, and digestive problems.

Senna (Cassia senna): This plant is used to treat a variety of health conditions, including constipation, fever, and respiratory problems.

Guanabana (Annona muricata): Also known as "soursop,"

this plant is used to treat a range of health conditions, including fever, cough, and digestive problems.

Neem (Azadirachta indica): This plant is used to treat a variety of health conditions, including skin problems, fever, and digestive issues.

African Basil (Ocimum kilimandscharicum): This plant is used to treat a range of health conditions, including fever, cough, and digestive problems.

Examples of Herbal Remedies Used in West African Traditional Medicine

West African traditional medicine is characterized by a wide range of herbal remedies, many of which have been used for centuries to treat a variety of health conditions. Some examples of herbal remedies used in West African traditional medicine include:

Fever remedy: A decoction of African Mango leaves is used to treat fever, while a poultice made from Neem leaves is used to reduce fever and alleviate symptoms. **Digestive remedy:** A decoction of Senna leaves is used to treat constipation, while a tincture made from African Basil is used to alleviate digestive problems.

Respiratory remedy: A decoction of Guanabana leaves is used to treat cough and respiratory problems, while a poultice made from Neem leaves is used to alleviate symptoms.

Challenges and Opportunities for West African Herbalism

Despite its rich cultural heritage and long history of use, West African herbalism faces a number of challenges. Some of the most significant challenges include:

Lack of formal recognition: West African herbalism is often not recognized by mainstream healthcare systems, making it difficult for traditional healers to access training and resources.

Limited access to plant material: Many of the plants used in West African herbalism are difficult to access, particularly in urban areas.

Cultural erosion: The cultural significance of herbalism is often being eroded by modernization and urbanization, leading to a decline in the use of traditional remedies.

Despite these challenges, there are also opportunities for West African herbalism to thrive. Some of the *most significant opportunities* include:

Integration with modern healthcare: There is a growing recognition of the importance of traditional medicine, including herbalism, in the treatment of a wide range of health conditions.

Conservation of plant material: Efforts are being made to conserve and protect the plant species used in West African herbalism, ensuring their availability for future generations.

Preservation of cultural heritage:

There is a growing recognition of the importance of preserving West African cultural heritage, including the traditional knowledge and practices of herbalism.

Herbalism in East Africa

Herbalism has been an integral part of East African cultures for centuries, with a rich history of using plants to treat various ailments and maintain overall well-being. The region's diverse flora has provided a vast array of medicinal plants, which have been used by indigenous communities to develop unique traditional healing practices.

Traditional Herbalism in East Africa

Traditional herbalism in East Africa is deeply rooted in the region's cultural and spiritual practices. Many East African tribes have a strong spiritual connection with nature, believing that plants have healing properties and are imbued with spiritual energy. Herbalism is often practiced by traditional healers, known as "waganga" in Swahili, who have spent years learning the art of herbal medicine from their elders.

In Kenya, for example, the Maasai people have a rich tradition of herbalism, using plants such as *"mukungu"* (Cassia abbreviata) to treat fever, and *"mwarobaini"* (Warburgia ugandensis) to treat snake bites. The Kikuyu people, on the other hand, use plants like *"muthi"* (Cassia occidentalis) to treat coughs and colds, and *"mugumo"* (Acacia tortilis) to treat skin conditions. In Tanzania, the Chagga people have a long history of herbalism, using plants such as *"kibuyu"* (Cassia obtusifolia) to treat fever, and *"mwarobaini"* (Warburgia ugandensis) to treat snake bites. The Zaramo people, on the other hand, use plants like *"mbuga"* (Cassia occidentalis) to treat coughs and colds, and *"mugogo"* (Acacia tortilis) to treat skin conditions.

Medicinal Uses of Herbs in East Africa

East African herbs have been used to treat a wide range of ailments, including fever, coughs, colds, skin conditions, and snake bites. Many of these herbs have been found to have antimicrobial, anti-inflammatory, and antioxidant properties, making them effective in treating various health conditions. For example, the "mukungu" plant (Cassia abbreviata) has been found to have antimicrobial properties, making it effective in treating infections such as pneumonia and tuberculosis. The "mwarobaini" plant (Warburgia ugandensis) has been found to have anti-inflammatory properties, making it effective in treating conditions such as arthritis and rheumatism.

Traditional Uses of Herbs in Southern Africa Herbalism

Southern Africa is deeply rooted in the region's rich cultural heritage. Each tribe and community has its own unique approach to herbalism, with a focus on the use of local plants and traditional remedies.

1. Medicinal Uses Herbs have been used for centuries in Southern Africa to treat a range of ailments, from minor injuries to serious diseases. For example, the Khoi and San tribes of South Africa used the roots of the *devil's claw plant*

(Harpagophytum procumbens) to treat back pain and arthritis. Similarly, the Zulu people used the leaves of the *wild garlic plant* (Allium ursinum) to treat respiratory infections.

Modern Applications of Herbalism in Southern Africa

While traditional herbalism is still an important part of Southern African culture, modern society is also beginning to recognize the value of herbalism in promoting health and wellness.

1. Integrative Medicine is a growing trend in modern healthcare, with many healthcare providers incorporating traditional herbal remedies into their practice. This approach recognizes the value of herbalism in promoting health and wellness, while also acknowledging the importance of modern medical science.

2. Cosmetics and Skincare Herbalism is also being used in the development of cosmetics and skincare products, with many companies incorporating traditional African herbs into their products. This approach recognizes the value of herbalism in promoting skin health and beauty.

3. Food and Beverage Herbalism is also being used in the development of food and beverage products, with many companies incorporating traditional African herbs into their products. This approach recognizes the value of herbalism in promoting health and wellness through diet and nutrition.

Modern Applications of African Herbs

African herbs have been an integral part of traditional medicine and cultural practices for centuries. The continent is home to a vast array of plant species, many of which have been used for centuries to treat various ailments, enhance beauty, and promote spiritual well-being. In recent years, the world has taken notice of the potential of African herbs, and their applications have expanded beyond traditional medicine to include modern industries such as cosmetics, pharmaceuticals, and agriculture.

9

Herbal Remedies in Latin America and The Caribbean

Discovering the Ancient Healing Secrets of Latin America's Forgotten Herbs

Latin America and the Caribbean have a rich and diverse cultural heritage, shaped by the indigenous, African and European influences that have coexisted and interacted over centuries. One of the most significant aspects of this cultural heritage is traditional herbal medicine, which has played a vital role in the health and well-being of the region's populations for centuries. The use of herbal medicine in Latin America and the Caribbean dates back to pre-Columbian times, when indigenous communities relied on plants to treat various ailments. The Mayans and Aztecs, for example, used plants to treat fever, rheumatism, and other diseases. The Spanish conquest of the region in the 16th century brought new plants and medical practices, which were incorporated into the existing traditional medicine.

African slaves, who were brought to the region, also brought their own traditional medicine practices, which blended with those of the indigenous and European populations. Cultural Significance of Traditional Herbal Medicine Traditional herbal medicine is deeply rooted in the culture and daily life of Latin America and the Caribbean. In many communities, herbal medicine is passed down from generation to generation, with knowledge and recipes being shared among family members and neighbors. Herbal medicine is often used in conjunction with other forms of medicine, such as Western medicine, and is seen as a complement rather than a replacement.

Types of Traditional Herbal Medicine

There are several types of traditional herbal medicine used in Latin America and the Caribbean, including:

Curanderismo: This is a traditional healing practice that originated in Mexico and is still practiced today. Curanderas use a combination of herbal remedies, rituals, and spiritual practices to treat a range of ailments.

Yerba Mate: This is a traditional medicine used in Argentina, Uruguay, and southern Brazil. Yerba mate is a type of tea made from the leaves of the South American holly tree, and is used to treat a range of ailments, including digestive problems and fatigue.

Bacrim: This is a traditional medicine used in the Caribbean, particularly in Jamaica and Haiti. Bacrim is a type of herbal remedy made from the bark of the guaiacum tree, and is used to treat a range of ailments, including fever, rheumatism, and skin conditions.

Uses of Traditional Herbal Medicine

Traditional herbal medicine is used to treat a wide range of ailments, including: **Digestive problems:** Herbal remedies such as *yerba mate* and *chamomile* are used to treat digestive problems, such as constipation and diarrhea.

Respiratory problems: Herbal remedies such as *eucalyptus* and *peppermint* are used to treat respiratory problems, such as bronchitis and asthma.

Skin conditions: Herbal remedies such as *aloe vera and chamomile* are used to treat skin conditions, such as eczema and acne.

Mental health: Herbal remedies such as *valerian root and passionflower* are used to treat mental health conditions, such as anxiety and insomnia.

History of Herbal Medicine

From pre-Columbian times to the present day traditional herbal medicine has been an integral part of the cultural heritage of Latin America and the Caribbean for centuries. From the pre-Columbian era to the present day, indigenous communities, African slaves, and European colonizers have all contributed to the development of this unique and rich tradition.

Pre-Columbian Era

(Before 1492) The use of herbal medicine in Latin America and the Caribbean dates back thousands of years to the pre-Columbian era. Indigenous communities, such as the Aztecs, Mayans, and Incas, relied heavily on plants and natural substances to treat a wide range of ailments. These communities developed sophisticated systems of medicine, often based on spiritual and mystical beliefs, which emphasized the interconnectedness of all living things. Some of the most commonly used herbs and plants during this period included:

Ayahuasca: A plant-based psychedelic brew used for spiritual and medicinal purposes, particularly among the indigenous communities of the Amazon rainforest. *Coca leaves:* Used for centuries by the Incas to treat a variety of ailments, including altitude sickness, pain, and inflammation.

Turmeric: A spice commonly used in traditional medicine to treat wounds, skin conditions, and digestive issues.

Colonial Era

(1492-1821) The arrival of European colonizers in the 15th century had a profound impact on the development of herbal medicine in Latin America and the Caribbean. African slaves, brought to the region against their will, brought with them their own traditions of herbal medicine, which blended with those of the indigenous populations. During this period, European colonizers introduced their own medical practices, often based on the teachings of Galen and Hippocrates. However, these practices were often ineffective in the tropical climate of the region, and indigenous and African herbal remedies continued to play a vital role in healthcare. Some notable figures from this period include: Francisco Hernández: A Spanish physician who traveled to Mexico in the 16th century to study the indigenous plants and medicines of the region. Juan de Torquemada: A Spanish friar who wrote extensively on the medicinal properties of plants in the New World.

Independence and Nationalist Movements

(1821-1945) The struggle for independence in Latin America and the Caribbean during the 19th century led to a renewed interest in traditional herbal medicine. As European colonial powers were pushed out of the region, local populations began to reclaim their cultural heritage, including their traditional practices of herbal medicine. During this period, nationalist movements and independence struggles often emphasized the importance of traditional medicine as a way to assert cultural identity and resist foreign influence. Some notable figures from this period include: José María Morelos: A Mexican revolutionary leader who advocated for the use of traditional medicine in the fight against Spanish colonialism. Antonio Saco: A Cuban independence leader who wrote extensively on the importance of traditional medicine in the struggle for national liberation.

Modern Era

(1945-Present) In the second half of the 20th century, traditional herbal medicine in Latin America and the Caribbean faced significant challenges, including the rise of modern medicine and the decline of traditional practices. However, in recent years, there has been a renewed interest in traditional herbal medicine, driven in part by the growing recognition of its potential benefits and the need to preserve cultural heritage.

Mexico

Mexico, a country rich in cultural heritage and biodiversity, has a long history of using herbal remedies and sacred plants in its indigenous cultures. From the ancient Mayans and Aztecs to the present day, Mexico's indigenous communities have relied on the wisdom of their ancestors to develop a unique system of traditional herbal medicine.

The Importance of Herbal Medicine in Mexico

Herbal medicine has played a significant role in Mexican culture for centuries. The country's rich biodiversity, with over 20% of its flora considered endemic, has provided a vast array of medicinal plants that have been used to treat a wide range of ailments. According to the World Health Organization (WHO), 80% of the population in Mexico still relies on traditional medicine, including herbal remedies, to meet their primary healthcare needs. Indigenous Cultures and Sacred Plants Mexico is home to 62 indigenous groups, each with their own distinct culture, language, and traditional practices. These communities have developed a deep understanding of the medicinal properties of plants, often using them in rituals and ceremonies to promote physical and spiritual well-being. Some of the most sacred plants used in indigenous cultures include:

Ayahuasca: A plant-based psychedelic brew used in shamanic rituals to communicate with the spirit world and access healing energies.

Peyote: A small, spineless cactus used in Native American Church rituals to induce visions and communicate with the divine.

San Pedro: A cactus used in Andean rituals to induce a state of trance and access spiritual guidance.

Tobacco: Used in traditional ceremonies to purify the body and spirit, as well as to honor the ancestors.

Traditional Herbal Remedies

Mexico's indigenous communities have developed a vast array of traditional herbal remedies, often using a combination of plants to treat specific ailments. Some of the most common remedies include:

Te de limón (Lemon tea): Used to treat colds, fever, and digestive issues.

Te de hierba (Herbal tea): Used to treat respiratory issues, such as bronchitis and asthma.

Susto (Fright): A traditional remedy used to treat anxiety, depression, and other mental health issues.

Mudanzas (Transfers): A traditional remedy used to treat physical and spiritual ailments, often involving the use of sacred plants.

Applications in Traditional Medicine

Mexico's traditional herbal remedies are used to treat a wide range of ailments, including:

Respiratory issues: Herbal remedies such as te de hierba and te de limón are used to treat respiratory issues, such as bronchitis and asthma.

Digestive issues: Remedies such as te de limón and te de hierba are used to treat digestive issues, such as diarrhea and constipation.

Mental health: Remedies such as susto and mudanzas are used to treat mental health issues, such as anxiety and depression.

Pain relief: Herbal remedies such as te de limón and te de hierba are used to treat pain and inflammation.

Brazil

Brazil, the largest country in both South America and the Latin American region, is home to an incredible array of herbal remedies that have been used for centuries. From the lush Amazon rainforest to the Afro-Brazilian traditions of the northeast, Brazil's rich cultural heritage is deeply intertwined with the use of herbs for medicinal, spiritual, and culinary purposes. The Amazon Rainforest: A Treasure Trove of Herbal Remedies The Amazon rainforest, which covers nearly 60% of Brazil, is one of the most biodiverse regions on the planet. The forest is home to an estimated 10% of all known plant species, many of which have been used by indigenous communities for centuries to treat a range of ailments. Some of the most commonly used herbs in Amazonian traditional medicine include:

Açai (Euterpe oleracea): A fruit that is rich in antioxidants and has been used to treat a range of conditions, including fever, diarrhea, and skin conditions.

Cat's Claw (Uncaria tomentosa): A vine that has been used to treat arthritis, rheumatism, and other inflammatory conditions.

Guarana (Paullinia cupana): A plant that has been used to treat fever, cough, and respiratory problems, as well as to increase energy and mental clarity.

Pau d'Arco (Tabebuia avellanedae): A tree that has been used to treat a range of conditions, including fever, cough, and skin conditions.

Afro-Brazilian Traditions

Herbal Remedies and Spiritual Practices Afro-Brazilian traditions, which originated in the 18th century, have had a profound impact on Brazilian culture and herbal medicine. Many AfroBrazilian communities use herbs to treat a range of conditions, including:

Susto (Fright or Shock): A condition that is believed to be caused by a sudden shock or fright, and is treated with herbs such as Guarana and Pau d'Arco.

Malandro (Syphilis): A condition that is treated with herbs such as Açaí and Cat's Claw.

Feitiço (Curse): A condition that is believed to be caused by a curse or hex, and is treated with herbs such as Pau d'Arco and Guarana.

Cuba

Cuba, an island nation in the Caribbean, has a rich cultural heritage that is deeply rooted in its history of colonization, slavery, and indigenous presence. This cultural melting pot has given rise to a unique blend of traditional herbal medicine practices that are distinct from those found in other parts of Latin America and the Caribbean.

African Influence

The transatlantic slave trade brought millions of enslaved Africans to the Americas, including Cuba. Many of these enslaved individuals were from the western coast of Africa, particularly from present-day Senegal, Guinea, and the Congo. They brought with them their own traditional herbal medicine practices, which were deeply rooted in their spiritual and cultural beliefs. In Cuba, African herbal medicine traditions were heavily influenced by the Yoruba people from present-day Nigeria. The Yoruba people had a rich tradition of herbal medicine, which was based on the use of plants, minerals, and animal products to treat a wide range of ailments. They believed that the natural world was inhabited by a multitude of spirits, and that the use of herbs and other natural substances could help to communicate with these spirits and restore balance to the body and mind. In Cuba, African herbal medicine traditions were often practiced in secret, as the Spanish colonizers sought to suppress the use of African spiritual practices. However, many African slaves continued to practice their traditional herbal medicine traditions in secret, often using the same plants and techniques that they had used in Africa. Spanish Influence The Spanish colonization of Cuba had a profound impact on the island's traditional herbal medicine practices.

Spanish herbal medicine traditions were based on the use of plants and other natural substances to treat a wide range of ailments, and were heavily influenced by the works of Greek and Roman physicians such as Galen and Dioscorides. Spanish herbal medicine practices were often based on the concept of "temperament," which held that the body was composed of four humors (blood, phlegm, yellow bile, and black bile) that needed to be balanced in order to maintain good health. Spanish herbalists used a wide range of plants and other natural substances to treat imbalances in the body's humors, and to restore balance to the body and mind.

Indigenous Influence

Cuba was also home to a number of indigenous peoples, including the Taino and the Ciboney. These indigenous peoples had their own traditional herbal medicine practices, which were based on the use of plants and other natural substances to treat a wide range of ailments. Indigenous herbal medicine practices in Cuba were often based on the concept of "sympathetic magic," which held that the natural world was inhabited by a multitude of spirits that could be communicated with through the use of plants and other natural substances. Indigenous herbalists used a wide range of plants and other natural substances to treat imbalances in the body's humors, and to restore balance to the body and mind. Evolution and Blending of Traditions over time, the African, Spanish, and indigenous herbal medicine traditions in Cuba began to blend and evolve. African herbalists incorporated Spanish and indigenous plants and techniques into their practices, while Spanish herbalists incorporated African and indigenous spiritual practices into their own traditions. This blending of traditions gave rise to a unique and distinctive form of traditional herbal medicine in Cuba, which was characterized by the use of a wide range of plants and other natural substances to treat a wide range of ailments. Cuban traditional herbal medicine practices were often based on the concept of "energetic balance," which held that the body was composed of a complex network of energies that needed to be balanced in order to maintain good health. Cuban traditional herbal medicine practices were also characterized by the use of a wide range of spiritual practices, including prayer, meditation, and rituals. These spiritual practices were often used to communicate with the natural world and to restore balance to the body and mind.

Modern-Day Practice Today

Cuban traditional herbal medicine practices continue to evolve and blend with modern Western medicine. Many Cuban herbalists have incorporated Western medical techniques and knowledge into their practices, while still maintaining their traditional herbal medicine traditions. Cuban traditional herbal medicine practices are also being used to address a wide range of modern health issues, including diabetes, hypertension, and cancer. Cuban herbalists are using their traditional knowledge and skills to develop new and innovative treatments for these conditions, and are working to integrate their traditional practices with modern Western medicine.

Jamaica

Jamaican folk medicine, including the use of bush teas and spiritual practices Jamaica, a small island nation in the Caribbean, has a rich cultural heritage that is deeply rooted in its African, European, and indigenous Taino influences. The country's folk medicine tradition, which is often referred to as "bush medicine," plays a significant role in the daily lives of many Jamaicans.

The History of Jamaican

Jamaican folk medicine has its roots in the country's African and indigenous Taino heritage. The Taino people, who were the original inhabitants of Jamaica, had a deep understanding of the medicinal properties of the island's flora and fauna. They used these natural remedies to treat a range of ailments, from fever and rheumatism to skin conditions and snake bites. The transatlantic slave trade brought African slaves to Jamaica, who brought with them their own traditional healing practices. African herbalism, which emphasizes the use of plants and other natural substances to promote health and well-being, became an integral part of Jamaican folk medicine. African slaves used herbs to treat a range of ailments, from respiratory problems to skin conditions. The arrival of European colonizers also had a significant impact on Jamaican folk medicine. European settlers brought